Lorraine Clissold lived in China with her husband and four children for ten years, between 1995 and 2005. During that time she learned to speak and read Mandarin Chinese, presented 'The Chinese Cooking Programme' on Central Chinese television, worked as a food writer and restaurant critic and set up The Chinese Cooking School from her home in the *hutongs* (narrow streets) of Old Beijing.

Now based in North Yorkshire Lorraine enjoys her family, her menagerie of animals, an outdoor life and home grown food. She spends extended periods in the French Alps, but goes back to Beijing for the best food in the world.

Lorraine is married to Tim Clissold, author of *Mr China* (published by Constable), whom she met when she was a student at Jesus College, Cambridge.

Find out more at www.chinesedontcountcalories.com

Why the Chinese
Don't Count Calories

Lorraine Clissold

CONSTABLE • LONDON

CONSTABLE
First published in Great Britain in 2008 by Constable,
an imprint of Constable & Robinson Ltd
This revised edition published in 2018 by Constable

A CIP catalogue record for this book
is available from the British Library.

ISBN: 978-1-4721-2766-2

Typeset in Bembo by Ellipsis, Glasgow

Printed and bound in Great Britain by Clays Ltd, St Ives plc

Papers used by Constable are from well-managed forests
and other responsible sources

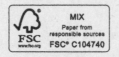

Constable
An imprint of
Little, Brown Book Group
Carmelite House
50 Victoria Embankment
London EC4Y 0DZ
An Hachette UK Company
www.hachette.co.uk
www.littlebrown.co.uk

To my grandfather, John Duncan Skinner

Contents

Acknowledgements

This book tells the story of my journey into a rich new culture. Were it not for my husband, Tim, I might still be sitting in Slough: thank you for everything you have done to support me in my work. Your passion for China and all things Chinese is infinite and I have been incredibly fortunate to have ready access to your expertise. Life as we have chosen to live it is not always easy, but nor is it ever boring.

My children kept themselves on course when my attention was directed elsewhere and even found time to help me out. Max was my own personal encyclopaedia; Christian was computer consultant and *mantou* chef all at once. Sam grew up when I wasn't watching and kept the animals fed and watered. Honor always had plenty to say about my cooking as well as questions about everything and anything. I look forward to having more time to share all your numerous interests as well as enjoying many more health-giving meals together.

My parents, John and Eileen, brought me up in a household where food is important (and always good) and have moved outside their geographical and culinary comfort zones with a spirit of adventure (sorry about the power cut in the *hutong* on Christmas morning), as well as providing an amazing level of emotional and practical support over the years.

Many of my friends in Beijing encouraged me to undertake this project. My thanks to everyone who attended the Chinese cooking school – I learned from you all. James and Lucy Kynge did a lot to build my confidence during my early courses; Faye Cowin was student and teacher alike; Fiona Key shivered cheerfully with me through many a lengthy dietary therapy class and helped me eat my way through many more extensive menus; Anne Wilbur kept me supplied with inspiring texts; Bettina Tioseco took some great photos; Lee-Ann Bissell was always prepared to listen; Linnet Workman gave her time generously to discuss my endeavours; Catherine Sampson was my inspiration as a writer.

Chinese food culture would not have been accessible to me had it not been for my patient and inspiring Chinese language teachers: T.C. Tang in London and Hong Yun and Wang Ye in Beijing. Professor Li of the Chinese Academy of Traditional Medicine helped unlock the secrets of Chinese food therapy and Professor Song of the Chinese Hospital of Traditional Medicine, provided an inspiring introduction to *Qi gong*. I have always found that the most interesting information is gleaned outside the classroom, and it is thanks to Feng Cheng of the Chinese Culture Club that I was introduced to Doctor Li Xin, whose individual approach helped me understand by own constitution and how to listen to my body and balance my diet accordingly.

I lived more closely with Ding Guo Ying (Xiao Ding) than with any other human being outside my own family and will always be indebted to her for both the direct and indirect ways that she shared her knowledge and experiences. Among my other Chinese mentors, Hao Min and Chen Bao Ling were particularly willing to share their time and expertise with me. Pei Pei Ren is as good a friend as one would find anywhere in the world, with that extra touch of Chinese kindness. Yu Tao Wang and Feng Ling taught me more than they will ever realize and I look forward to watching my godchild Silas flourish in a multicultural society.

While we were overseas friends and family back in Europe did a lot to maintain our connection with our previous life. My sister Amanda Rose has shared her knowledge of food and nutrition and has always been there for me and the children. Debbie and Mark Loveday have been the best friends anyone could ask for; Nicki Carmichael has been supportive throughout; Rowan Pees has been a motivating force in my life; Bridget Tracy found time in her hectic schedule to read some early writings. Maurice and Neena Pellier, Gilles Baltazar, Renee Roulet and Sebastian Broel have helped us all so much in France. Rebecca Ellis has been my lifeline in Yorkshire.

Special thanks to my agent, Toby Eady, and Xinran whose interest in my work has continued since that first Chinese meal in our draughty courtyard home. I am grateful to Nick Robinson at Constable & Robinson for his faith in me and to Andreas Campomar and Eleanor Dryden for leading me through the daunting business of publishing. Celia Hayley provided invaluable direction, support and encouragement throughout the editing process. I thoroughly enjoyed sharing my experiences and ideas with you all.

This list is not definitive. The fifteen years since I first set foot on Chinese soil have been filled with fascinating encounters with interesting people from all corners of the world. Snippets of conversations overheard in the street, throwaway comments in local restaurants, the pertinent observations of taxi drivers and lively discussions in my cooking school, have all contributed to the richness of the experience which I bring to my readers. With thanks to all those who made it possible, I present a personal and individual interpretation of a fascinating subject; any misapprehensions or errors are my own.

Lorraine Clissold
April 2008

Note on the use of Chinese characters

The pinyin style of Romanization is used throughout this book, except for words and names that are in common use in other spellings. These include Taoism, Confucius, Mencius and Tai Chi.

Recipes

Serving Suggestions

Figures and tables

Prelude

I first went to Beijing in the summer of 1993. Before this, my experience of Chinese food was limited to the Golden Panda, a cheerful place on the top level of the shopping precinct in the small Sussex town where I grew up. I had fond memories of prawn toasts, crispy seaweed, and spring rolls served on oval platters. We would choose a set meal, which unfailingly featured glossy strips of lemon chicken, soggy orange balls of sweet and sour pork, sticky red spare ribs, salty silvers of black bean beef and a token of mixed vegetables, based on tinned beansprouts. If we opted for Set Meal D, we would get a few battered king prawns and there would be a handful of shrimps in the 'special' fried rice. I especially looked forward to the jelly and ice-cream served in sundae glasses. Anyway, the the food on these occasions was very much secondary to the idea of a night out and working it all off on the dance floor to the sounds of 'Sugar Baby Love' and 'Saturday Night Fever'.

So I did not set out for China's capital with any great expectations on the culinary front. In fact, as I stepped onto the burning tarmac of Beijing City Airport, food was not much on my mind. I was at a crossroads in my life and needed to move forward, and when a voice from my past proffered an invitation to visit the East, the opportunity to exchange my pedestrian existence as a single mother of two young boys in Slough for a touch of freedom and romance was too good to miss.

My relationship with Tim, which had started in the heady days of university life, floundered in our twenties as different aspirations put thousands of miles between us. Friends and family warned me sternly of the dangers of rekindling an old flame, but I wanted to see what had captured Tim's heart. For two glorious weeks I allowed myself to revel in the incessant activity of Asia's fastest-growing capital, keeping irregular hours, letting each day unfold as it might and opening my senses to a culture that both beckoned and intimidated all at once.

With Tim's help I acquired a Flying Pigeon bicycle, the brand favoured by all the locals, inappropriately named, I thought, since it neither went very fast nor knew its way home. It did, however, allow me easy access to the narrow streets, known as *hutongs*, where I could savour the sights, sounds and smells of local life. Occasionally I would visit a park or a temple, but, perhaps because I am by nature a home-maker, I increasingly found myself drawn to the street markets and the food stalls. There, the throngs of local Beijingers were all united in a common purpose, which appeared to be a routine but not a chore, and the city really came alive for me.

Early morning was grocery time. I was amazed by the sheer volume of foodstuff, most of it green, much of it unrecognizable, that could all be loaded on a three-wheel cart. People shopped with energy and enthusiasm, often entering into lengthy exchanges that I guessed must be about price or quality. Stallholders would willingly offer to break open a tomato to show the succulent flesh or peel back the silk of a sweetcorn to display the fresh cob inside. I watched with interest to see a surly man attack a radish-type vegetable with a chopper and reveal a bright purple centre; I held my breath as a cheeky-faced young girl smashed a green egg, exhaling only when I found out that the contents were solid and bright orange in colour.

Some people say that dog owners come to look like their animals; I couldn't help making the same comparison between the vendors and their produce. A women selling tomatos had had round smooth rosy cheeks, a clear-skinned girl with perfect features offered me a succulent grape to try; a small shy man with close-cropped hair sat shelling peas; a tall thin youth peered over piles of what I first thought were leeks, but later discovered to be spring onions. A weatherbeaten type sold unwashed carrots and potatoes and an octogenarian sat scooping up walnuts and dates into paper bags. 'Even the rugged and wrinkled look fit,' I thought to myself as the old man's face broke into a smile, which crinkled his skin like a piece of thin paper.

When my stomach announced that lunch-time was nearing, I was irresistibly drawn to the multitude of street snacks in hole-in-the-wall outlets or on portable trolleys. The sweltering August weather provided a steamy backdrop for slurping huge bowls of noodles, but this was no deterrent for the locals. Most tables had a bamboo tray or two with some kind of steamed bun or dumplings that the diners grasped deftly with their chopsticks, dipped into a dark liquid, and expertly devoured in two bites. I would walk past them slowly, attempting to get a closer look at what they were eating, without attracting their notice or staring too hard. Sometimes I couldn't help but stop in amazement at the vibrance of the scene, and when I did I noticed that young and old and very old, well-dressed, casual and downright shabby were all represented among the street-side clientele. Yet despite obvious disparaties of age and income the diners had many things in common: healthy countenances, shapely physiques and sheer enjoyment of the moment.

Not a natural communicator and totally lacking in language skills, I was often frustrated in my attempts to sample the local flavours. While I had read about intrepid travellers dining in fine style just by pointing; I did little more than cope, and wasn't comfortable interacting. I was far too worried about attracting attention to myself, being cheated, robbed, or simply laughed at. I was also concerned about what I might end up with. Would it be greasy and inedible? Would I be obliged to eat it anyway?

Alone on my first day in Beijing, I made my way past every stand in the street, convincing myself that the food at the next one would be better, or the ordering process clearer, but ended up in the Beijing Hotel, safe in the company of the city's affluent tourist population. There I ordered a tuna sandwich, which bore little relation to its name.

Realizing that I had to do this in stages, I turned my attention away from the hundred-and-one varieties of noodles and the mysterious bamboo baskets towards more recognizable items. By the end of my first week I had managed to buy a couple of small fried flat-breads. The filling was still a lottery: flat chives with flecks of egg, an aniseed-flavoured vegetable with minced pork, or, sometimes just minced spring onion. I did feel vaguely guilty about the amount of oil that oozed from my prize, and the vegetable was vaguely reminiscent of grass cuttings, but the whole eating experience was much better than the tuna sandwich, so I put my misgivings aside.

In the early evening (even in 1993 restaurants in Beijing seldom stayed open after eight), we would go slightly up-market on the eating establishment front. During the ten years that Tim and I had spent apart he had acquired an enviable level of spoken and written Mandarin, which opened a wealth of possibilities. Laughing at my inability to decipher even the

simplest of Chinese characters, he taught mc to identify restaurants by the string of fairy lights outside or the tank of fish
within and to favour places where we had to squeeze in among
the cheerful locals and avoid those where a lone waitress sat
watching TV or slept with her head on the plastic tablecloth.
Then, waving aside the extensive handwritten menu, Tim
would order confidently from his repertoire of favourites.

The dishes we ate in Beijing, seated at rickety wooden
tables on folding chairs, bore no resemblance to the Golden
Panda's set menu. On my first night we ate in what can only
be described as a shack, which we approached across a building
site. After showing me how to rinse my slightly grimy glass
with water from the kettle before pouring my beer, Tim ordered
three dishes. I remember each one clearly: a plate of chicken
and peanuts, with whole dried chilies in view, an aubergine
dish featuring some kind of mushroom and, finally, glistening
bright green mange-tout peas with a liberal scattering of garlic.
It looked like a lot of food for two people, and I had a rather
lightweight pair of disposable chopsticks to deal with, not to
mention misgivings about the whole chilies and the fungus;
but the smell was so tantalizing that I dug in manfully.

The chicken dish, Tim's favourite, *gong bao ji ding* (which
masquerades in the UK as 'Kung Pao chicken', see p. 109) was
more than spicy: it totally filled my mouth with heat. I thought
I had experienced the ultimate taste sensation until I tried the
aubergine. This was slightly hot, with a hint of sweet and sour
too, and an usual flavour that I later learnt was fermented bean
paste. The sauce lingered on the pieces of fungus, which were
surprisingly firm to chew, contrasting well with the soft chunks
of aubergine. My chopstick skills proved a match for everything,
even the flat thin crisp mange-tout, which were so much more
appetizing than the rather grey-green string vegetable I was

familiar with. Before I knew it the plates were empty and we were fighting for the roughly chopped pieces of garlic left on the oval plate.

As we emerged into the balmy street, I looked around me. There were at least six similar establishments within sight, all packed and certainly not with the rich and famous. In China, I realized at that moment, good food is accessible to all. I asked Tim to stop for a moment and we peered into a neighbouring restaurant. Against the soothing background of a brightly lit fish tank the atmosphere was animated and the diners looked totally at ease, digging eagerly with their chopsticks into an amazing variety of dishes. 'These people just love their food,' I thought to myself, and then another thought followed quickly in its wake: 'but not one of them is overweight'. That is not to say that everyone had supermodel proportions: the shapely took their place alongside the skinny and the rounded contrasted with the thin, without anyone looking uncomfortable or out of proportion. The night was warm, and on a couple of tables the the beer was flowing, but where cheeks were flushed it was with rude health, not overindulgence.

As we strolled through the balmy night Tim gave me a quick insight into the Chinese food culture. 'Accept the fact', he explained in the affectionate tone he always uses when describing anything China-related, positive or negative, 'that they're obsessed with food. . . . There is a whole set of rules for formal eating. Sometimes it can take ten minutes just to get everyone seated at the table so that no one takes offence.'

I made a mental note to avoid formal dinners. 'But what about everyday eating?' I asked, thinking fondly of the lively atmosphere we had just witnessed. Tim explained that when he listened carefully, he found that the conversation usually revolved around food. 'Mealtimes are major events in China;

people think and care about food all the time. Food is ingrained in their culture,' he said, 'the meals are the high points of the day.'

'Obsessed with food!' I turned the phrase over in my mind. I could relate to that. I had spent most of my college years planning what I would cook my friends for supper, the result being a great following from the opposite sex but a second-rate degree. Then I had found myself a job in food PR writing catchy copy lines like 'our sausages contain no eyeballs nor snout' and producing recipe booklets for low-calorie salad dressings. My enthusiasm for the subject was such that I had been prepared to spend hours in photo shoots making coffee look frothy with a splash of washing up liquid or painting tomatoes with glue to make them glisten. I even once toured the country with a dinosaur costume arranging tea parties for the winners of a competition on cans of dinosaur-shaped pasta pieces. Once the actor missed the train and I found myself walking the streets of Hull with a gaggle of children hanging onto my tail, which stretched my enthusiasm for the job to the limit – but didn't quench my enjoyment in working with food.

The problem was that my food obsession was tinged with a trace of guilt. Part of the first generation to be plagued with modern, lifestyle-related obesity, I grew up in an era of fad diets and obsessive calorie counting and had seen several of my contemporaries suffer from anorexia. So, convinced that restraint was the only option, I was fascinated to come upon a nation that positively stuffed at every meal and looked great on it. I could see that the Chinese obsession with food was different.

One sweltering afternoon I emerged from the dining room of the China World Hotel. Some of Tim's colleagues' wives had invited me to lunch, and I had had my first experience of an American-style buffet table. The meal had been unexciting: greasy red noodles, dried up pieces of barbecued meat and shaving foam-topped gateaux. According to habit I had helped myself from the selection of rather tired looking salads and was leaving the dining room feeling distinctly dissatisfied.

As I hit the street, a tantalizing smell wafted from a doorway. The door was ajar and I couldn't resist a look; perhaps it was the kitchen? Even better – it was the staff dining area. The noise and activity were a sharp contrast to the sophistication of the hotel restaurant. I couldn't help but notice the quantity that people were eating; their rice bowls were not the dainty cup-sized ones that I was familiar with but big enough to toss a salad in or serve pasta for two or more. And they were full with a multi-coloured, multi-textured teetering pile of food. I recognized a waitress from the hotel dining room; she had introduced us to the sumptuous display of food with an air of efficiency and politeness that lightly masked her disdain. Now, sitting with her head down, bowl in one had, chopsticks in the other she was totally at ease. As she came up for air, I caught her eye and held it. She smiled. At that moment I knew that she, and thousands of others, had secrets to share, and I determined to find them out. It took me ten years, and I am still learning.

By the summer of 1995, I was fully in pursuit of real Chinese food. Married to Tim, I had completed a Mandarin course and was living in Beijing with my two sons, Max and Christian, then aged six and four, and our new baby, Sam. I took every opportunity to frequent local restaurants and order as many different dishes as possible. That was the easy bit, and fortunately the boys enjoyed the multitude of new tastes and flavours and the relaxed atmosphere where children are not just welcomed but positively doted on. Adjusting to a culture where it is usual to have an *ayi*, or home help, was more diffi-cult, but, over time, I came to appreciate the arrangement for the great privilege that it is. Two years my senior, fresh-faced and slim with waist-length hair, our *ayi*, Xiao Ding, did not take long to become an integral part of our household and we are firm friends to this day. Xiao Ding gave me invalu-able practical assistance when I arrived knowing no one in an alien capital city and although neither teaching me the secrets of the Chinese kitchen nor helping me set up a cooking school formed part of her original job description, she rose to the challenge and provided guidance and inspi-ration throughout.

I knew that a good working knowledge of the Chinese language was the only way to unlock restaurant and kitchen doors, so I set about to further my Mandarin studies with a vengeance, baby seat in tow. Chinese, while relatively simple in terms of grammatical constructions, seems completely impen-etrable at first sight since every new character has to be learnt by rote. But necessity is a great motivator, and I was soon able to get myself around town and feel comfortable in restaurants and in the markets. Chinese cuisine appeared equally daunting at times, as there were dozens of ingredients that I had never seen before. I would wander round food stores in a daze, trying to make sense of row upon row of bottles, piles of packets filled with pastes of some kind and bags of dried produce that might have been animal, vegetable or mineral.

As I made progress in the language my teacher began to reward me by finishing the lesson with a menu or a recipe to translate. Then I found a book with the riveting title of *Chinese Vegetables*. It had some rather bad line drawings with names in English that were often wrong and in the full form

Chinese characters used in Hong Kong and Taiwan, with pinyin (alphabetical pronunciation) for the Cantonese dialect, which meant nothing to me because it is used only in the south of China. My Chinese teacher, Wang Laoshi, was patient and supportive. She led me through the pages, discussing the many uses of the different vegetables and writing in the Mandarin pinyin pronunciation of the names. After class I would walk home through the vegetable market proudly armed with my new knowledge. In the evening we would feast on delicacies: sliced red radish with green peas and minced ginger, silken squash with egg and pork slivers, *you mai cai* (rather like cos lettuce) with fish and black bean, or homemade pancakes stuffed with beansprouts, egg and Chinese chives. With every new discovery and every successful dish I felt my relationship with food underwent a subtle change, a change for the better. I became the controller, not the controlled, and these changes were a source of great pleasure to me. My obsession with food had tranformed from a fixation to a passion and I was slimmer, fitter and more at ease with my body than ever before.

Three years and a baby daughter, Honor, later my hard work was rewarded when a colleague of Wang Laoshi put me forward for my dream job: presenter of Chinese Central Television's Chinese cooking programme. 'We need someone who knows a little about Chinese food, can read sufficient Chinese to translate recipes from Chinese to English and speaks enough of the language to chat and joke with the chef on the set.' I was open-mouthed as I heard Wang Laoshi tell her that I would fit the bill perfectly.

My learning curve was probably steepest during the CCTV years, but the knowledge it armed me with was well worth the pain of extraction. My producer, Hao Min, had ideas about how Chinese cooking should be taught to the home-cook that were right in line with mine. We would start with an ingredient and then show the audience how to use it. More often than not the main ingredient was a vegetable. 'Please talk for five minutes about celery,' Hao Min said, expectantly, on my first day. I was horrified, but so touched by her faith in me that I didn't tell her that I had anticipated a script running across the wall in front of me neatly out of sight of the cameras. It was bit like a party game. I said a little prayer of thanks for my years spouting PR, to Wang Laoshi, to my vegetable book and to my ability to remember obscure bits of information, particularly when related to food. Holding out the rather limp Chinese variety of celery (*qin cai*) in a gesture that later caused hilarity among my family and friends, I pointed out that it has a much better flavour but a shorter shelf-life than the stiffer, crunchier thick stalks known in China as *xi qin* or American celery. Quite truthfully, I explained that I had rediscovered celery in the interesting combinations of my favourite Chinese dishes.

The transition from TV presenter to teacher in my own cooking school two years later was a natural one. I loved learning from Hao Min and the chefs but wanted a greater degree of control over the content of my presentation and a closer interaction with my audience. By then I had come to believe that there was a lot more than recipes to be learned from Chinese food culture, and I knew how many westerners in Beijing were curious to learn more about Chinese food; so I set about putting together a suitable course to teach them. The establishment of the Chinese Cooking School was a not-insignificant project that involved much hilarity in the kitchen and fun in the marketplace, but also hours of recipe-testing and many a late night at the computer.

During the four years that I spent teaching westerners to cook Chinese food I became increasingly aware of both the vast differences between the eastern and western food cultures and the potential for bridging this gap. I was privileged to be able to discuss food and diet with such a large number of interested individuals from all over the world. My students came with varying expectations: some wanted little more than to enjoy a Chinese meal in the company of friends; others hoped to learn to decipher restaurant menus; but a significant minority shared my desire to gain a deeper understanding of the way that Chinese people shop, cook and eat. Whether or not they actually intended to wield a chopper and stir a wok themselves, they all wanted to eat more Chinese food. Those who discovered that a good Chinese diet can be enjoyed on a daily basis without any reservations, or the tedium of calorie-counting that has become the norm in some cultures, went away satisfied in more ways than one.

I was fortunate to live in China in the 1990s, when the food culture was still largely untouched by western influence. Sadly, this is not still the case, as multi-nationals fight to win the palates and strip the pockets of the world's largest market. Changing lifestyles and the power of marketing have begun to influence eating patterns in some parts of urban China and resulting obesity and diet-related health issues are now being acknowledged. History has shown, however, that Chinese culture is so strong that, in the long term, it is able to withstand invasion, and those who have conquered China usually come round to the Chinese way of doing things. My belief is that China's food culture is so strongly ingrained that it will ultimately remain largely as it has been for thousands of years; my hope is that as eating habits and patterns of consumption become increasingly globilized its benefits will be recognized and it will influence the rest of the world.

While the fifteen secrets I reveal in this book are those of traditional Chinese food culture, and though along the way I introduce the Chinese way of shopping, preparing food and cooking as well as many new and unusual ingredients, it is not necessary to eat a totally Chinese diet in order to benefit from the knowledge I have to share. Since we returned to live in the UK in 2005, I have had neither regular access to specialized ingredients nor the luxury of Xiao Ding's expert guidance. With four children and a small menagerie of animals, I sometimes struggle to find time outside my domestic and chauffeuring duties to make and serve nutritious meals. But what I brought with me from China and what I present here is not just about new recipes, although I have included some for you to enjoy. It is about crossing a cultural boundary to discover a different way of thinking about food and diet. If you can make this transition you will find that your desire to eat well and your understanding of how to prepare good food will propel you through even the most hectic periods of your life with new energy and vigour.

During my time in China I developed a new and exciting relationship both with food and with my own body. I acquired an understanding of the cuisine and host of skills that allowed me to produce satisfying and nutritious meals for my family and pass my knowledge on to hundreds of students. But that was not all. Food is just one aspect of the rich and varied Chinese culture. *Zhong guo* (China) literally means Middle Kingdom: the largest population in the world has survived political and geographical upheavals by pursuing balance in all areas of life and and avoiding extremes.

Over the years my studies moved on to the fascinating area

of Chinese food therapy, a branch of Traditional Chinese Medicine (TCM), based on the Taoist theories of the Five Elements/Phases and the opposing forces of *yin* and *yang*, which dominate Chinese thought and are explained in the Chinese Classic the *Yi Jing* or 'Book of Change'. Using these theories as their basis, Chinese doctors have observed human beings and recorded, refined and consolidated their findings for more than 3,000 years.

As I delved deeper into Chinese philosophy and came to understand the 'middle way' of the Tao of Laozi, I began to realize that a good diet is not a panacea but just one important part of a way of life that keeps mind and body fit by respecting the natural order of things. The parting words of Professor Song, my *Qi Gong* teacher, have stayed with me, and it is in the spirit of these words that I present these Fifteen Secrets:

> Take what you have learned, practise it, adapt it as necessary, and make it work for you. Then, when you are ready, take the time to teach someone else.

one

Stop counting calories

——

'When you eat you should not worry.'
SUN SI MIAO (581–682 AD)

One of the first things Tim told me about life in China was how he had spent the first year of his time there bemused by a girl who asked him every afternoon whether or not he had eaten yet, even though he had told her in the first week that he never ate lunch. Eventually he realized that the phrase '*Ni chi fan le ma?*' ('Have you eaten yet?') is just a way that people greet each other in in China.

This simple sentence, with its mixture of concern and interest, says a lot. Eating is important in China; food is not a matter for concern and worry but a source of great pleasure. Chinese people get pleasure out of every aspect of food, from planning or anticipating a meal, through preparing or choosing various dishes, eating and enjoying them and considering the meal in retrospect.

Chinese people talk about *yingyang*, the nutritional value of food all the time. There is a word for calories, *re liang*, but it is a scientific term (literally meaning 'measure of heat') and scarely understood by lay people. When I was weaning my son, Sam, Xiao Ding was quick to suggest that I feed him on puréed carrots rather than potatoes because they had more *yinyang*. Fascinated, I quizzed her carefully and found that, though she had never heard of calories, or vitamins and minerals for that matter, and because she grew up during the Cultural Revolution, had had no formal education, she had firm ideas about which foods were good to eat and in what combinations.

During that brief conversation over a bowl of puréed potato, I learned the first secret of Chinese food culture: think about food as something that will nourish you, not as a source of unwanted calories. In my mind, before I went to China, food was something that made you fat, unless you were very careful. Those who openly enjoyed eating seemed to have resigned themselves to a future of elasticated waistbands and an early death. The only alternative was constant vigilance. At only five foot two and a comfortable size ten, I was often dubbed 'lucky' by my larger friends. But there was no luck about it. As a first-year student, heady with the freedom of university life, I had eaten and drunk with the best of them. After six months of canteen food, sausage rolls, chocolate bars on the run and crisps in the pub, I had gained nearly a stone in weight – not disastrous but certainly very noticeable on my small frame, especially when some supposedly concerned friends marched me into Woolworth's and put me on the scales. It had taken six weeks working in a campsite in the south of France and a strict regime of fruit and salad to get back to my former size. The heat, coupled with the physical labour of daily tent-cleaning, not to mention the need to wear a bikini around all those handsome French youths, helped me in my resolve.

From that summer on, periods of pregnancy aside, I started to watch my weight carefully. I would lie in bed at night and where I had once recited the Lord's Prayer, I would run through the calories I had consumed that day. As I was looking to maintain weight rather than lose it, and I have a tendency to remember such useless information as how many calories there are in a digestive biscuit, this was a simple exercise to perform. Breakfast was usually branflakes with skimmed milk and wholemeal toast with a scraping of something; lunch was never more than a sandwich or a salad. By keeping my daytime intake to around 800 calories I could allow myself a reasonable evening meal, perhaps a pasta or chicken dish, even a curry, and a couple of glasses of wine. If I ever topped my 2,000 calorie-a-day limit I would compensate the following day. By sticking to these rules I was acceptably thin. Okay, I drunk endless cups of tea and coffee to keep hunger at bay and I was often quite ratty by early evening; I also suffered a range of minor ailments like headaches after eating, bloating, poor digestion and varicose veins, and I was constantly exhausted – but the doctor said that it was all pretty normal. Sadly, he was probably right. Many people in the West have a compromised relationship with food and many more suffer from a host of nagging discomforts; and the general feeling is that these problems are a bit like bad weather, something we have to live with, and be thankful for the sunny days.

I once met a former anorexic who religiously ate a Kit-Kat for lunch on the basis that it contained only 120 calories and therefore fitted neatly into her self-imposed allowance of 1,000 calories a day; but she would never dream of eating a portion of potatoes, rice or pasta with a similar calorific intake because they were 'fattening foods'. Another time I sat through an extremely expensive six-course meal in a London restaurant with a girl who showed me how she had acquired the art of messing around with her food to make the waitress think that she had eaten some of it. The aim of the exercise, she confided, was to save her calorie allowance for the chocolate mousse, *petit fours* and truffles. Our western obsession with calorie-counting has created a whole raft of new issues: anorexia, bulimia and other forms of malnutrition. Millions of pounds are spent on special dietary formulas, hours are wasted on slimming classes; in hospitals, surgeons are wiring jaws and stitching stomachs.

After my conversation with Xiao Ding I took a closer look at the products on sale in the Chinese stores. In 1995 in China there was no such thing as a pre-prepared meal, breakfast cereals had not made their appearance and there were a limited number of biscuits and confectionary products on the shelves alongside the Chinese staples of grains, nuts and dried fruits. I scoured the packaging carefully: not a single calorie count did I find. A nightmare, I thought, for anyone on a 'WeightWatchers' programme. But then, I realized, no one was. Chinese people will pontificate for ages on the health bene-fits of different foods, sharing knowledge that has been handed down through the generations, and will often make quite personal remarks about how a person needs to eat more of one type of food than another; but no one would ever consider the value of a food in terms of its calorie content. Food in China is enjoyed because it looks good, smells good, tastes good and does you good. And the people that I saw all around me were obviously benefiting. China has no special clothes shops for the 'fuller figure' or special facilities for large people. When I lived in China, obesity simply wasn't an issue. In 2002 in a multi-cultural study on attitudes to body shape, children from different countries were shown silhouettes of figures ranging from very thin to obese. While American children viewed the very obese figures as their least preferred shape, Chinese children had no negative feelings about obesity; it appears that they didn't believe such fat people existed.[1]

We don't know what to eat

The year I arrived in China and was marvelling at the wealth of foods in the Chinese diet, a Mass Observation survey in the UK found that 'society now relies almost completely on convenience foods. Working people start the day with a bowl of cereal and milk and sugar, and drink tea; throughout the day they eat biscuits and sandwiches and drink more tea; once at home, few of them seem to cook a meal for themselves from raw ingredients.' This picture is very bleak, and numerous campaigns have improved the situation in recent years, but it does explain why western dieters often end up by starving themselves. Cut out the bread and biscuits that have been pinpointed as 'baddies' and what is there left to eat? Manufacturers have had a field day producing low-fat, low-calorie versions of the limited number of foods that western consumers feel comfortable with: diet yogurts, low-fat biscuits, sugar-free drinks, butter substitutes, oil-free salad dressings. The Meat Marketing Board has produced leaner pigs; the dairy industry has taken the fat out of milk. We have spent the last few years hung up about what not to eat, when there are thousands of foods out there packed with nutrients, but we don't know what to do with them.

How easy is it to put aside all the baggage of western nutrition speak, when the 'count your calories' message is screamed at us from the packaging of our 'healthy' breakfast cereal, throughout the day in shops, in magazines and on the television and, for many, last thing at night as we fill in our WeightWatchers chart? Until I saw the Chinese way of eating with my own eyes I did not really believe that it might be possible to enjoy food without guilt, and without getting fat.

In the West we have been indoctrinated with the idea that the only way to lose weight is to eat less and exercise more. During my first year in Beijing I went to a talk organized by the International Newcomers Network (INN). The speaker was the fitness instructor from the leisure centre at a leading hotel: the message was 'join our gym and you will never have to worry about your weight again'. Not yet immune to the western mindset, and with new-found leisure time thanks to round the clock domestic help, I joined. I even found a driver to take me there. I tended to exercise in the late morning while my youngest was asleep and leave during the lunch-time rush as the place filled up with sweaty businessmen. On my way out I would glance into the canteen to see a bunch of drivers enjoying a slap-up lunch. And I couldn't help but consider that, despite the fact that some of them had to cycle to and from their place of work morning and night, generally a driver's lifestyle is pretty sedentary – and I didn't see many fat ones.

I was slightly envious of the camaraderie that was so evident in the Chinese canteens. While I was puffing away in silence on the running, step or rowing machines, watching the counter record the energy I was burning, all the Chinese staff, from the manager to the receptionist and the waitresses to cleaners, were enjoying a feast with friends. My reward for burning off an extra 200 calories might be an extra slice of slightly stale bread with my salad and a digestive biscuit for tea: but was I really any better for it?

I am not disputing that exercise does burn off calories or that restricting food intake can help lose weight. What I question is a food culture that has allowed these principles to take away the pleasure of eating, which traditionally was a positive experience associated with nourishment, good health and sustaining life.

At this stage you will undoubtedly be thinking that there *must* be a catch. The West *is* getting fatter and we all know that this is because we are taking in more calories than we burn off. So, if the Chinese do not need to count calories yet manage to stay slim and fit, is there a genetic or lifestyle factor involved? Or perhaps, despite the appearance of eating a lot, are they actually eating a low-calorie diet because of the types of food in their diet?

All these questions went through my mind, too. My quest to discover the secrets of the Chinese diet was originally totally unhampered by any scientific training or method; my only qualification was my enthusiasm for the subject and a burning desire to understand why the West's relationship with food has gone so terribly wrong. Modern science, with all its strengths, tends to concentrate on single factors; I wanted to understand a whole culture and was as interested in unquantifiable factors such as attitudes to food as I was in comparative calorific intake and obesity levels.

The Chinese eat more calories

As my understanding developed, I found many of my observations vindicated by modern research. Chinese people do actually eat more than westerners and yet stay thinner. *The China Study* by T. Colin Campbell claims to be 'the most comprehensive study of the link between diet and disease ever published'. A survey carried out by Dr Campbell and a world-class scientific team in 1990 questioned 6,500 adults from sixty-five counties across China and compared the statistics with those gathered in different countries, particularly the United States. Not only did the survey result in 8,000 statistically significant associations between lifestyle, diet and disease but it had 'startling implications for weight loss'. Any investigation into eating habits necessarily includes a record of calorific intakes and bodyweight. *The China Study* showed that when Chinese were compared to Americans: 'The average calorie intake, per kilogram of bodyweight, was thirty per cent higher . . . Yet bodyweight, was twenty per cent lower.'[2]

Chinese people eat more calories than Americans, but keep slimmer – extraordinary. 'So the Chinese must be more active!' you will cry with relief, and resolve to use that gym membership. Certainly when they saw the local people stuffing themselves with huge portions of food three times a day, my

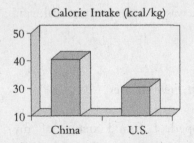
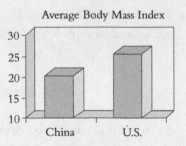

1. **Calorie consumption and body weight**[2]
(Courtesy of Campbell and Campbell, *The China Study*.)

western friends were generally quick to assume that the Chinese don't worry about counting calories because they need to fuel their active lifestyles. And indeed most Chinese people still live and work on the land, and those living in towns will generally walk or cycle to work. But what about all the sedentary drivers enjoying their huge lunches? Or the Chinese scholastic tradition and the hundreds of thousands of office-bound civil servants?

The *China Study* team ranked the Chinese into five groups according to their activity levels: the figures above relate to the least active group of Chinese (the sedentary office worker) compared to average Americans (moderate exercise several times a week).

The Chinese are not thinner because they take in fewer calories or because they take more exercise. 'Then it must be in the genes,' you will conclude with resignation. (People claimed to have 'heavy bones' when I was a child; now 'a slow metabolism' is more fashionable.)

The gene theory is tempting, but too simplistic. With different ethnic backgrounds come different lifestyles and eating habits. It is easier to point to the one thing that cannot be emulated than find out more about those that can; but, over the years, I have been fortunate to be able to delve behind skin colour and into lunch-boxes.

Before moving to Beijing I took a Mandarin course in London. In the early stages of my third pregnancy, I entered my first class with a touch of trepidation, not to mention nausea. I couldn't tell if the other students were in a gap year or recent graduates, but their fashionably grubby clothes exuded the enthusiasm and self-assurance of youth. It was with enormous relief, therefore, that I noticed Paula sitting alone and took up a seat beside her. Like about half the class, Paula was ethnic

Chinese, but whilst the others were mainly the children of Cantonese restaurateurs, focused on the career opportunities that the language of the motherland could offer, Paula was a wife and mother, and more interested in rediscovering her roots. United by age and responsibility, we became firm friends within the week.

On the first day we soon left the smoke-filled common room and ventured into the concrete expanse of the town to eat our lunch. As I suffered the hunger pangs that I considered par for the course in pregnancy, I noticed that Paula, whose petite stature made me feel quite gargantuan, never tried to get by on a sandwich at midday. Her lunch-box revealed a mound of rice topped with meat and vegetables. I watched in disbelief as her fingers worked the chopsticks. This was no midday snack, yet she was talking excitedly of the meal she would cook that evening. Whilst her family may have neglected to maintain her linguistic heritage, their culinary legacy was obviously still intact – and she looked great on it.

Ladies who lunch (and don't get fat)

The first friend I made when I arrived in Beijing was May, the wife of one of Tim's colleagues. May was from Hong Kong and loved to 'lunch'. It was at her apartment, with its panoramic view of the Sanlitun Embassy district, that I had my first real taste of Chinese home-style cooking. Eating with May and her friends from Taiwan, Singapore and Malaysia was confirmation that throughout the whole of Asia people eat well; they positively celebrate food and never talk about restricting what they eat in any way. We would take steaming bowls of rice or noodles and top them with a selection of tasty morsels. I discovered the delights of lotus root, fibrous and delicate in flavour, and stem lettuce, crunchy and tasting slightly of asparagus, and I began to recognize the fermented bean pastes that give so many Chinese dishes their distinct flavour and to distinguish one type of beancurd from another. They introduced me to foods I didn't know existed, like the delicately filled tiny parcels of Cantonese *dim sum*, crisply wrapped Japanese sushi, Korean noodles that blew my head off and the fascinating flavours of the local stir-fries. I also learned that there is more to aubergine than ratatouille and far more to cabbage than bubble and squeak. When these women talked about food it was with excitement and pleasure. While the bias of their diet was towards freshly cooked savoury dishes they did not have any taboos or no-go areas. When the school bake sales came round, which they did with monotonous regularity, they could produce a cheesecake or a plate of muffins that would rival Betty Crocker.

May and her Asian friends were all slim, despite the fact that eating was their favourite occupation. Like Paula, they all appeared to have been been brought up in households with a positive attitude to food. But during my time in Beijing I also had plenty of opportunity to observe other Asians, whose eating habits had been influenced by western ideas or lifestyles. Those of ethnic Chinese heritage who are born in the West are loosely described in Asia as American-Born Chinese (ABCs). As China's economy boomed in the 1990s thousands of ABCs were attracted back to the home of their ancestors. One of these was my friend Deborah, a British-Chinese doctor, whom I met during a routine consultation and who had an enviable command of self-taught Mandarin that I hoped might open some restaurant doors for me. Solidly built to the extent that her white coat was stretched across her stomach, she certainly looked as if she must enjoy food.

I met Deborah for lunch. She ordered nothing but a water-melon juice; I invited her for supper and she picked at her meal complaining of a stomach upset. She seemed to live on air, and despite our initial spark I never became close to her. When we met at social functions I continued to notice that, despite her size, she never seemed to show any interest or pleasure in food.

So what about the 'thin gene' theory? Deborah, like May and Paula, was ethnically Chinese and all three were from similar socio-economic backgrounds. Yet while two of my friends loved to eat, and ate a lot, the third avoided the subject whenever possible. Yet it was Deborah who had the weight problem. She was not in control of her eating; she was over-weight and unhappy.

Three case histories do not make a statistic, but studies have shown that adolescent obesity increases significantly among second and third generation immigrants to the United States.[3] Time spent in my children's international school confirmed my suspicions. Among the ABC children, who almost outnum-bered the others, obesity and other related problems, such as bad skin and allergies were common; and these children were often fussy eaters or on self-imposed diets. Yet the hordes of tracksuit-clad local Chinese youngsters who thronged the streets in the early morning and evening, looked slim, fit and bursting with health. And they did not pick at their food or choose low-calorie options. My oldest son, Max, spent a year in Number 55 Middle School, a local public Chinese school, when he was thirteen years old. I gave him 3 RMB (about 25p) a day, which bought him, like his classmates, a bowl of rice and accompanying dishes. On his first day he ate tomato and egg, pork with carrot and bamboo shoots, and stir-fried *xiao bai cai* ('little white cabbage', which is actually green), with chilli. He never came home hungry.

My years of living and eating in China and everything I learnt and taught has led me to conclude that the first and fundamental difference between the way people eat in China and in the West is one of attitude. Instead of seeing food as an enemy and focusing on what not to eat, often depriving the body of nutrients, the Chinese focus on making food taste good and meeting the body's needs. It does not occur to Chinese people to approach food with trepidation, or to worry that the occasional treat will lead to unwanted pounds and inches. The Chinese eat more calories but not the 'empty calories' full of fat and sugar and devoid of all nutrients, which make up a high percentage of the western intake.

Never a day passes by in China when you do not hear the phrase 'Have you eaten yet?' Focus on the fact that more than a billion people in China, and millions more in Asia, eat regularly, eat a lot, and never worry about counting calories – and put your hang-ups aside.

two

Think of vegetables as dishes

—

'As long as one has the art, then a piece of celery or
salted cabbage can be made into a marvellous delicacy.'

YUAN MEI (1716–98), NOTES ON HIS COOK

In the very early morning and in the evening, when Chinese
people flock to the colourful food markets that suddenly
appear on every corner, they pass each other in the street with
the greeting '*Ni mai cai qu?*' ('Are you going to buy vegetables?').

It was one of my Chinese teachers in Beijing, Hong Yun,
a slender young graduate from Bei Da University, who enlight-
ened me about Chinese greetings. She was explaining how
Chinese people greet each other. The quaint phrase '*ni hao*'
(literally, 'you good') means hello, but the Chinese use a variety
of phrases depending on the time of day or the situation. 'Have
you eaten yet?', as we have seen, is the usual acknowledge-
ment around lunch-time. A man passing a neighbour on the
way to work usually greets him with, 'Are you going to work?',
to which the reply is, 'Going to work,' spoken in a grunting

sort of way, with a 'humph' at the end. In the late afternoon a similar exchange: 'Are you going home?' is answered by 'Going home, humph.' So Chinese people start the day with a trip to the *zao shi* or early morning market, and they say '*Ni mai cai qu?*' ('Are you going to buy vegetables?').

The Chinese character *cai* (vegetable) also means a dish of food. Understand this and you will have unearthed the second, and possibly the most important, secret of the Chinese diet. When I first noticed the two uses of the word *cai* I assumed that I had made a mistake. Chinese is tonal, which means that when a word is pronounced with a flat tone, or with an upward inflection, or an up-and-down inflection, or a downward one, it has completely different meanings even though it sounds very similar to the untrained ear. The confusion between the spoken word, the tones, and the underlying Chinese characters is the biggest challenge for the student of Chinese, and even sometimes the Chinese themselves.

The *cai* that means vegetables is pronounced with the same downwards inflection as that which means a dish of food. Some Chinese words are pronounced the same but written differently, but *cai* is written in exactly the same way, whether it is used to describe a vegetable in the generic sense or a dish of cooked food. Most Chinese characters are split into two parts, the first part, known as the radical, often gives a clue to the meaning of the word, while the remainder of the character might hint at the pronunciation. *Cai* has the grass radical, signifying that it is something that grows, while the the lower part of the written character is indicative of the *ai* (pronounced 'I') sound.

Living among the Chinese and witnessing the tricycles overflowing with greenery, and the locals returning from the market every morning with their loaded bags soon makes it clear that this double meaning is no coincidence. And sampling Chinese vegetable dishes confirms the fact that vegetables can be a meal in their own right, with small amounts of protein foods used to add interest.

This is not to say that the Chinese do not eat meat: on the contrary, meat tends to be prized and valued, and there is no part of animal, fish or fowl that a Chinese chef cannot turn into a feast. The everyday diet, however, is based for the most part, around vegetable dishes.

Frequent visitors to Chinese restaurants or readers who have travelled in Asia may find this difficult to believe. Restaurants make their name and higher margins on meat and fish dishes and, because the same animal species are available across the globe whereas vegetable varieties vary greatly, the restaurant tradition has evolved this way. Most famous Chinese dishes are protein-based because these are the recipes that are usually recorded and passed on. Added to this, meat has a longer shelf life than most plant varieties, and is not seasonal. In ordinary Chinese homes, however, vegetables form the main dishes. Worthy of the same treatment as meat and fish, they are carefully prepared with slicing or dicing, interesting seasonings and accurate cooking times and they are never served as a hasty afterthought, chopped roughly or boiled to death.

If you were a child of the sixties as I was, you might well have been brought up on vegetables cooked in a pan of salted water, boiled until soft, if not reduced to a total pulp. Prepared in this way vegetables never stand a chance of playing anything other than a poor supporting role. Recently the West has rediscovered vegetables. In the UK, the 'five a day' campaign has taken hold and of course vegetables feature heavily in weight-loss plans, whether cabbage soup, low GI and GL, or just good old calorie restriction. One reaction to the problems that have resulted from an increasingly limited diet in the West is for a number of gurus to recommend 'super' or 'bonus' foods. Next time you pick up one of the excellent books on nutrition now on offer, take a look to see if it has a list of foods with protective properties or exceptional nutritional value. They always make me smile, since nearly all the foods they recommend are daily fare in China.

Vegetables, as we now know, are the 'good guys', packed full of the vitamins, minerals and active constituents that were previously overlooked in the macronutrient approach of western experts which emphasized protein, carbohydrate and fat and played lip service to vitamins. A portion of frozen peas, a glass of orange juice, a handful of vacuum packed salad leaves all help us notch up that 'five a day' total. Food manufacturers have relabelled all their products to draw attention to the number of vegetable portions they contain and are busy launching new nutrient-packed vegetable substitutes too. We are making a tremendous effort to get vegetables back on the stage; but in China they have always been in the limelight.

In China the 'bonus foods' of the new 'healthy' western diet are not taken as supplements, or served as token seasonings or side dishes. Onions are stir-fried with lamb, not lamb with onions; celery is served with strips of beef, not beef with celery. Green chilies are shredded and mixed with coriander and cucumber in the aptly named *laohu cai* ('tiger dish'); sometimes chilies are just stir-fried with more chilies. Ginger and garlic are thrown into recipes by the fistful; there are 101 recipes for cabbage and aubergine.

The difference between the quantities of vegetables bought, used in cooking and eaten in China and the West is difficult to visualize. The first time I saw root ginger stacked up on a hessian mat at the side of the street I assumed it was Jerusalem artichoke: I had never seen more than a couple of pieces in western supermarkets and here it was piled waist high. Soy beans and mung beans were another source of amazement: a small market would sell a two-foot mountain in one day, more, I reckoned, than the weekly turnover of my local supermarket in the UK.

When the stallholders in the Chinese markets noticed a 'foreigner' they would excitedly hold out tomatoes, lettuce, potatoes, carrots and, on a good day, broccoli. Dismissive of these imports, but more influenced than I realized by nights at the Golden Panda back home, initially I would search for baby corn (not sold in northern China), water chestnuts and bamboo shoots (both seasonal and unrecognizable anyway in their unpeeled state); but gradually I simply learned to choose what looked good and fresh.

How to transform the *cai* in the market into the deliciously presented *cai* on Chinese tables was not something I learned overnight. On the contrary, I spent many an hour pondering this problem – when I should have been doing my Chinese homework.

Culinary barriers are always difficult to penetrate. I knew that to discover the secrets of the Chinese diet I needed to learn to cook. This is a difficult concept to communicate, especially to someone to whom the art is obvious. My first efforts to tap Xiao Ding's store of knowledge were disastrous. One day I braved the market and bought some ingredients that I considered 'Chinese': beansprouts, mange-tout and some very watery pink-looking prawns. She was not impressed. Dismissive of the prawns she simply took the beansprouts and fried them with Sichuan peppercorns, minced ginger and spring onion, and some fresh red chilli, and then tossed in some chopped coriander. A splash of vinegar on the beansprouts keeps them crisp. Soy sauce, she explained should be avoided as it makes them brown and soggy: a pinch of salt is used instead. No cook worth his salt – or even his soy sauce – would want to detract from the beansprout's greatest attribute, its crispness. After she had washed and dried the wok she chucked in the mange-tout and fried it with a generous handful of garlic and a good pinch of salt. I could not believe that such a delicious dish was so simple to prepare.

I soon discovered that Xiao Ding could make a dish out of any leaf, shoot, root or tuber that I chose to bring home, but that she generally liked to take one ingredient at a time and choose a method and seasoning that cooked it to perfection. Sometimes two ingredients that complement or contrast each other are put into the same dish, but they are usually cooked separately and mixed together at the last moment. Thin shreds of meat or tender morsels of fried egg are often used in dishes where vegetables take the leading role. The strips are made tender by coating them with cornflour and treating them with a drop of cooking wine. Or beaten eggs are added to hot oil in the wok, then stirred with chopsticks to break them into pieces as they puff up.

A new look at familiar vegetables

Working with Xiao Ding and eating in local Beijing restaurants completely transformed my attitude towards even the most mundane of vegetables.

Cabbage
Take cabbage, which was the bane of my school dinners as a child, but which is something of a national obsession in China.

At one time, in northern China, the large Beijing cabbage, known as *da bai cai* ('big cabbage'), which is usually sold abroad as 'Chinese Leaves', was practically the only leafy vegetable available. Fortunately this humble vegetable is bursting with vitamins and the anti-oxidants which are now being shown to fight the damaging effects of free radicals, so it was able to provide even the poorest country-dwellers with a substantial supply of nutrients.

In 2001, the average Beijing resident consumed 77 pounds of cabbage.[4] As a comparison, the highest ever consumption of cabbage in the US was in the 1920s (22 pounds per capita); the 2003 estimate was 7.5 pounds.[5] When I was first in Beijing the government still handed out free supplies of cabbage in urban areas, organizing blue 'Liberation' trucks to rumble in from the countryside so that people could fill their courtyards and balconies with enough to see them through the winter. In 1989 the supply outstripped demand and the government urged people to eat up the stocks, earning Beijing's favourite vegetable the name of 'patriotic cabbage'. The outsides sometimes got frostbitten, but the tight-packed leaves inside remained crisp and fresh for months. Young, comparatively affluent people like my teacher Hong Yun were slightly embarrassed by this state generosity, seeing the cabbage as a reminder of an unhappy past, but I saw how many old folk and families were grateful for the gift. And there is no doubt that most Chinese people like cabbage — as would most people if they knew how best to cook it.

The Chinese name *bai cai* means 'white vegetable', and the ubiquitous *da bai cai* (big cabbage) is light in colour. But Chinese chefs can also choose from *xiao bai cai* (small cabbage), *yuan bai cai* (round cabbage), *Shanghai bai cai* (Shanghai cabbage), *naiyou bai cai* (milk cabbage) and *ta cai* (rosette cabbage). And there are a host of other greens: *you cai* (rape vegetable), the amusingly named *jimao cai* (chicken feather vegetable), *tong hao* and *haozi ganr* (Chrysanthemum leaves), *you mai cai* and *gan lan*, which have no western names to my knowledge, and various types of spinach and watercress too. While I have not seen many of the more esoteric varieties for sale in the West other than in ethnic stores, we have picked shoots of wild rape from our local farmer's field after the major crop (which is used as animal fodder) has been harvested. Chinese leaves are pretty commonplace in the West and the popular 'sweet-heart cabbage' is similar to the Chinese round cabbage in its cooking qualities. *Xiao bai cai* is increasingly available in super-markets, sold under the Cantonese pronunciation of its name, *pak choy*. In the spirit of Chinese cooking, though, I have used many of our alternative brassicas and leafy greens, including curly kale and good old greens, in Chinese-style dishes.

While only a handful of the vegetables varieties that are enjoyed in China are readily available in the West, the truth is that what you may or not be able to buy is not a fraction as important as what you are able do with it. All the white cabbage varieties are greatly enhanced by a touch of ginger and chilli or sweet and sour seasonings. Dried chilli spices up both the green and the white types and can also be used with western spring greens or kale. Cabbage needs to be well cooked, until the leaves wilt, but overcooking makes the flavour too strong. Cumin can add a depth of flavour and helps digestion.

Stir-fried cabbage in China is often complemented by reconstituted dried Shitake mushrooms or wood-ear fungus. To this strips of pork may be added, but with cabbage they should not be coated in cornflour or flour as this would clog up the clear sauce that seeps out of the cabbage leaves. Peeled

Chinese cabbage with red chilli
(La bai cai)

辣
白
菜

This dish is best made with the large cabbage usually sold as 'Chinese leaves' and sometimes as 'Peking cabbage' in the West, but other types of cabbage can be used. In the winter these cabbages are piled up in almost every court-yard and balcony, so this is the Chinese equivalent of a 'store cupboard' dish.

1 small Chinese cabbage (about 500 g/1 lb)
2 dried red chilies, roughly chopped
1 tsp finely chopped ginger
1 tsp finely chopped spring onion
1 tsp light soy sauce
1 tsp vinegar
½ tsp sugar
½ tsp salt or to taste
1 tbsp oil

Chop the cabbage into pieces of about 2 cm (1 in) square. Using gloves, crumble the dried chilies. Heat the wok, add the oil and heat to a medium heat. Throw in the chilies and let them sizzle but not burn.

Turn up the heat and add the cabbage, ginger and spring onion. Toss and fry, keeping the cabbage moving so that it cooks quickly and evenly (long handled chopsticks are best for this task). As the cabbage starts to soften, add the vinegar and sugar and stir-fry for another minute. Add the soy sauce and the salt, stir, turn down the heat, and simmer for another minute or so (liquid should seep out from the cabbage at this stage, creating a moist and flavoursome dish). Remove from heat and serve immediately.

chestnuts go very well with white cabbage varieties, especially with a touch of sugar and vinegar.

Mushrooms

Mushrooms are another vegetable whose potential is not always fully tapped in the West. For many people the white button variety is synonomous with the whole species and is often relegated to the role of a garnish in cooked breakfasts or used in soups and sauces. Chinese markets have whole stalls devoted to different varieties. The most common is *xiang gu* (fragrant mushrooms), a delicacy in the West where they are known by their Japanese name, Shitake. Freshly picked and piled high they take their place along with oyster mushrooms, straw mushrooms, *enoki* mushrooms, chestnut mushrooms and an amazing species known as 'chicken leg' because that is exactly what they look like. There are also separate stalls devoted to dried mushrooms (of which Shitake is the best known) and fungus of all shapes and sizes that promise a sensational flavour experience. Studies show that Shitake mushrooms may have anti-cancer properties. Keen to benefit, adventurous western cooks are adding a few to risottos or mushroom soup, but the cost of using them in any quantity is prohibitive. Yet mushroom recipes abound in Chinese cooking. One of the simplest ways that Shitake mushrooms are served is stewed with ginger and soy sauce as a dish in their own right. The Yunnan region in the south-west is renowned for its mixed fresh mushroom stir-fries, the north-east uses dried varieties heavily in stews and hot pots. The most expensive and best quality dried mushrooms, large *dong gu* (winter mushrooms) are used in a recipe with slices of large winter bamboo shoots in a dish called *chao er dong* ('stir-fried two winters').

More and more mushroom varieties are becoming available

in the West; in particular I love the large field mushrooms. Don't wait till you find a recipe for a specific variety; as with cabbage, the different types are quite interchangeable – or you can cook several types together. Mushrooms are very quick to prepare and suitable for any meal occasion. I stir-fry them with onions and herbs and serve them on toast, in an omelette, with rice or pasta or with a green vegetable such as asparagus, spinach or green beans – and they are delicious curried with lentils, or topped with a creamy paprika sauce, or with breadcrumbs and herbs. Garlic, of course, is a natural partner for all mushroom varieties, though ginger works well, too

How to 'eat your greens'

The Chinese are adept at turning simple vegetables into taste-filled dishes. The simple bromide 'eat your greens' has echoed down the generations in the West, but leafy green vegetables are also among the worst victims of bad or excessive cooking, all too often added to a meal as an afterthought and eaten in sufferance. Pay them the attention they deserve, however, and they will respond to even simple treatment with delicious flavours.

One of the most common ways that Chinese chefs cook simple green leafy vegetables (including lettuce) is *suan rong*, with minced garlic. The wok is heated and a good tablespoon of oil added. Then the vegetables are thrown in and tossed about until the the leaves begin to wilt. A sprinkling of salt and as many as six cloves of minced garlic are added and mixed thoroughly. More fibrous vegetables, such as broccoli florets, can also be cooked in this way but they need to be blanched first: the pieces are thrown into a pan of boiling water, brought back to the boil, then drained. Ideally, the

Braised mushrooms
Lu xiang gu

The word *lu* is often translated as 'flavour potted' and usually describes an aromatic broth in which the ingredients are marinated. In this instance, though, the broth is quick and simple to make – but delicious nevertheless. This dish is best served cold, though not chilled.

75 g/3 oz/¾ cup Shitake mushrooms
a few slices of ginger
1 tsp light soy sauce
½ tsp sugar
¼ tsp salt (or to taste)
pinch of white pepper (optional)
warm water
1 tsp sesame oil
1 tbsp oil
1 tbsp chopped coriander

Soak the mushrooms overnight (or, if you forget, 15 minutes in boiling water will do). When they are soft, cut off the stalks then check the underneath for any small particles of grit and rub clean. Rinse and drain.

Heat the oil in the wok to a medium temperature. Fry the mushrooms with the ginger pieces until they change colour. Add the soy sauce, sugar, salt and pepper to taste. Pour in just enough water to cover the mushrooms. Simmer for five minutes or so, topping up the water if necessary, until the mushrooms are plump and soft.

Turn off the heat, add the sesame oil and mix gently. Allow to cool. When ready to serve, arrange the mushrooms cap side up on a plate and tip any remaining sauce over the top. Garnish with chopped coriander.

drained vegetable is plunged into ice-cold water before stir-frying; this helps to retain the bright green colour.

'White' vegetables

Similarly, 'white' vegetables like potatoes or courgettes do not have to be thought of as bland or uniform foods. Chinese chefs manage to make some of the least interesting vegetables into the most tasty of dishes. Potatoes, courgettes and daikon (white) radish, for example are shredded into matchsticks then tossed in the wok over a very high heat with ginger and spring onions, Sichuan peppercorns, and/or crumbled dried red chilli, sugar and vinegar, a splash of soy sauce and a pinch of salt. Cumin can work well with the radish too, as it does with cabbage. After the first few thorough tosses, the heat is turned down and the liquid seeps out of the vegetables to form a delicious sauce with all the nutrients still in place. Salt is always added last; otherwise it can spoil the colour of the dish and detract from, rather than enhance, the flavour.

Delicate flavours

Some vegetables are prized in China for their own delicate tastes, and these are served freshly cooked and very lightly seasoned. Bamboo shoots, which are available in many different shapes and sizes depending on the time of year they are picked, are particularly treasured. Fresh water chestnuts and baby corn need little additional seasoning. Bear this in mind if you have access to freshly picked ingredients; a sprinkling of salt and a good quality oil may be all that you need to bring out their intrinsic qualities.

In Chinese cooking the oil carries the flavour while the salt, added tactically at the last moment, along with other seasonings, adds the depth of taste needed to let the vegetables carry the meal. If you begin to eat lightly cooked vegetables on the scale that they are consumed in China, and let them replace the processed and prepared foods in your diet, you won't need to concern yourself with your fat and salt intakes – believe me.

Chinese people have based meals around vegetables for thousands of years and have perfected the art of cooking them. Not a meal is served without steaming great plates of freshly picked and freshly cooked greens (and lots of other colours too). As we have seen, you can follow Chinese recipes to enliven your vegetables, or use more familiar methods to make them into dishes your own way. Every cuisine has its share of vegetable recipes, it is just that they are too often included in cookbooks as an afterthought, and our western mindset regards them as such. Following the restaurant tradition, cookbooks tend to deal with the various animal species first, then perhaps look at eggs and cheese and finally bring in the greens. Sometimes vegetable recipes are so simple that they are not taken seriously. But everyone appreciates a lightly-seasoned-tender steak, so why not give the same consideration to asparagus, carrots or even cabbage?

Just as the Chinese use small shreds of meat or fried egg in stir-fried dishes, or a piece of fatty lamb to flavour a stew, so you may chose to use small amounts of cheese and cream, as well as the more familiar herbs and spices, to make your vegetables tasty and interesting. Milk products are not much used in traditional Chinese cooking, largely because of economic

菜 ## Simple ideas for Chinese Style *cai*, or vegetable-based dishes

Stir-fry

with minced garlic:
blanched broccoli • spinach • asparagus • courgettes • all mushrooms • mange-tout • lettuce

with dried chilli and Sichuan peppercorns or cumin seeds (add rice vinegar and a pinch of sugar for sweet and sour touch):
shredded cabbage (all varieties) • beansprouts • daikon radish (with carrot) • shredded potato • greens • courgettes • kale

with ginger, spring onion, and shreds of meat (optional):
boiled green beans • beansprouts • courgettes • celery • onions • green pepper • tomatoes

with ginger spring onion and stir-fried egg:
spinach • tomatoes • cauliflower • aubergine (with tomatoes) • cucumber • sliced and boiled flat beans (add a few strips of bacon too if desired) • wood-ear fungus

Steam or boil

top with sesame oil and soy sauce, salt or oyster sauce:
green beans • broccoli • carrots • baby corn • celery • asparagus • pumpkin and other squashes

Boil

and top with olive oil and salt (and fresh herbs, crushed walnuts or olives):
beans • broccoli • spinach • new potatoes • brussels sprouts (top with grated lemon rind and ginger)

and mash with nutmeg or garlic:
pumpkin • parsnip • carrot • beetroot • mixed root vegetables

Stew

with Indian spices or coconut and chilli:
pumpkin • beetroot • cauliflower • potato • mixed vegetables

in tomato sauce with herbs or cumin:
red and yellow peppers • aubergine • courgette • cauliflower • finely chopped mixed vegetables

Bake

blanched and stuffed with a rice or grain based mixture:
peppers • onions • aubergine • courgette • flat mushrooms (no need to blanch)

sliced with onions:
potato • courgette (and tomato) • aubergine • celeriac • sweet potato

factors (China, for the most part, does not have good pasture-land, so it would have had to import dairy products) rather than dietary preference. Instead, as we shall see later, they have a large number of soy-based products, the multitudinous health benefits of which are only just being discovered in the West.

While not everyone has ready access to bountiful street markets and few of us live in extended families where there is always someone on hand to help with the shopping and cooking, we do have some advantages when it comes to preparing interesting vegetable recipes. Well-stocked super-markets make it possible to plan ahead; modern western kitchens boast fridge-freezers, and ovens have built-in timers. You can stick a bake in the oven, throw together a vegetable curry or stuff some courgettes or peppers. With a multi-dish approach (see Chapter Four) and with your new appreciation of everyday vegetables you might fry a mixture of fresh and soaked dried mushrooms with garlic, make fresh tomato sauce, grill some aubergine slices or make a purée of sweet potato and carrot. Make your transition to the Chinese style of eating gradually, and your delicious vegetable dishes will soon take over the meal without your having to arrange a *coup*. Before you know it you will find yourself eating a healthier, more interesting and surprisingly satisfying diet.

three

Fill up on staple foods

三

'*Qiaofu nan wei wu mi zhi chui.*' ('Even the cleverest housewife cannot cook without rice.')

OLD CHINESE PROVERB

The Chinese language can be very literal, but occasionally it is extremely imprecise. The word *fan*, as in '*Ni chi fan le ma?*' ('Have you eaten yet?'), is used in this context to mean food, or a meal. But the precise translation of *fan* is rice, so in fact what people ask each other every day is 'Have you eaten rice yet?' Just to add to the confusion, though, rice, in this context, means 'staple food', not only 'rice'. In China a meal is not a meal without a substantial element of *fan*.

The essence of a Chinese meal, the *fan* and *cai* concept, where vegetable-based dishes are partnered with a staple such as rice, is an ingrained part of Chinese culture: records show that the concept existed in the Shang dynasty around 1500 BC. Western nutritional science, as such, dates back not much more than 100 years. Wilbur Atwater, known as the father of American nutrition, worked hard to secure public funds for his food investigations in 1894. In the UK glaring deficiencies in the diet of urbanized societies were acknowledged between the world wars. The first published surveys recommended that starvation should be kept at bay with sufficient supplies of bread, fat — mainly butter and margarine, potatoes and oatmeal. Ironically, it seems that when people started to get fatter rather than fitter the finger was pointed to the same foods.

In Beijing, the food culture is traditionally wheat-based, and noodles or *mantou* (steamed buns) are popular *fan* for many. In the northern countryside people eat millet, which is very nutritious but not versatile, since it does not cook into separate grains. Cornmeal, currently fashionable in the West under its Italian name 'polenta', was once considered the staple of peasants, but tasty cornmeal cakes and flat breads are now enjoying a revival in Beijing's nostalgia restaurants. Even lower down the staple ladder is the starchy sorghum (the Chinese name *gao liang* translates as 'tall millet') which can grow in the driest of agricultural areas and is therefore regarded as a poverty food. Today sorghum is used mainly for fermenting into vinegar, while the stalks, a source of sugar, are also used for firewood or even as a wattle-like building material. Potatoes are generally viewed not as *fan* but as a vegetable to be made into *cai* (I have enjoyed many a meal of potatoes with rice); Chinese farmers were too astute to treat such an unreliable crop as a staple.

Without *fan* it is impossible to *chi bao* ('eat until you are full'), as Xiao Ding made very clear to me when she accompanied us to the UK one summer. We were enjoying a traditional roast lunch at the home of some friends. I was aware that the whole performance was a struggle for her and noticed that when she put down her knife and fork with what sounded like a sigh of relief, she looked at me for guidance. I asked her if she would like any more beef or vegetables? Or roast potatoes perhaps? Away from Beijing my Chinese sounded pretty good, especially as only Xiao Ding had the faintest idea what I was saying and she had a vested interest in understanding me, stranded in this totally alien environment.

'*You fan ma?*' she asked. At first I thought she was saying, 'Is there any food?' and was stumped for a moment. But I was not the only one who was confused; Xiao Ding elaborated on her previous question: '*Dou shi cai,*' ('It's all dishes'), she explained. '*Mei you fan ma?*' ('Is there no rice?'). I suddenly realized what she meant. Xiao Ding, who was slight even by Chinese standards, had already amazed our hosts by feasting heartily on slabs of roast beef, accompanied by generous servings of brussel sprouts and boiled carrots, with at least four roast potatoes; but now she wanted to know where the rice was.

Trying to explain to Xiao Ding how, in the West, meals usually consist of meat and two veg and that we break down our diet into proteins, carbohydrates and fats stretched my Chinese to the limit. I don't know how much she understood, but I could see she had no intention of being fobbed off with potatoes as *fan*. In the end I made her a couple of peanut butter sandwiches, as our hosts stood by open-mouthed.

In a Chinese meal *fan* is usually a substantial portion of a rather plain staple. From a culinary viewpoint, it serves as a foil for the highly flavoured *cai* and, of course, it fills you up. Dumplings are an exception since they combine both *fan* and *cai*, though they are placed in the *fan* category, illustrating the superior importance of the staple. The simple dumpling wrappers are made of a flour and water mixture with little or no seasoning, so as to provide a bland partner to the tasty filling, in a microcosm of a full Chinese meal.

When we eat Chinese food at home I give everyone a bowl of rice and we put morsels of food on to it so that the rice can soak up the delicious sauces. In restaurants, however, the rice or other staple is generally served last. Restaurateurs prefer to hold back the cheap filling staple for as long as possible to encourage guests to order the expensive *cai*. This change of emphasis might be a treat for people on an evening out, and has helped perpetuate the myth that the Chinese diet is based on rich protein-based dishes, but no one eats like that in China on a regular basis.

I have spent many an hour poring over menus in local Chinese restaurants. Chinese people love to put things in categories and feel strongly about agreed definitions. A usual menu will always include *liang cai* (cold dishes), *re cai* (hot dishes) and *zhu shi*, which literally means 'the most important food' and in common parlance is described as *fan,* the staple. Very few waiters will question a diner's selection of *cai* no matter how random it appears to be. But if a guest is unfamiliar with the Chinese way of doing things and omits to order the *zhu shi*, the waiter will hover expectantly and eventually point out the omission. No less than one portion of *zhu shi* per person will be deemed sufficient.

There is no doubt that in the Chinese food hierarchy, *fan* comes way above *cai*. Western nutritionists introduced the 'food pyramid' with its base of carbohydrate foods more than 3,000 years after the Chinese had worked out that a diet based on a staple food made economic, environmental and nutritional sense. In times of scarcity *fan* was eaten on its own, and people survived. Even today it is acceptable to eat *fan* without *cai*, or a staple without dishes, but not to eat *cai* alone, as it seemed to Xiao Ding I had expected her to do.

During my first years in China, I used to slip back into

western eating patterns on our annual trips to the UK. I exchanged my Chinese-style lunch for the chilled ready-made soups, pre-packed salads and the offerings of the local butcher's delicatessen counter. It took about a week before Xiao Ding started to make herself huge bowls of noodles topped with whatever vegetable was cheapest in the local greengrocer. As I struggled to find interesting foodstuffs for her to use I realized how the protein-centred approach of the average modern-day western meal makes for very limited eating.

A steaming bowl of rice, on the other hand, offers endless possibilities for interesting accompaniments to those who know how to prepare them. Rice is considered the superior staple in China from an economic, nutritional and culinary view-point and, except in areas where necessity has forced populations to become accustomed to another grain, is generally favoured. In Europe we are just beginning to widely appreciate the many benefits of this versatile, natural, non-allergenic and easily digestible food, but very few people eat it on a regular basis. Unlike bread, rice does not lend itself to eating away from home or 'on the run' (although the Chinese have got round this problem with steel lunch-boxes). As the carbohydrate element of a main meal it is unlikely to be eaten more than a couple of times a week, especially in a food culture where carbohydrates have had years of bad press.

The western food culture's modern-day fear of *fan* has not been helped by the protein-loaded Atkins and South Beach diets, or the idea of food 'combining', where proteins and carbohydrates have to be eaten at different meals. Restrictive eating plans of this kind may be effective in the short term, generally because they result in the dieter eating less overall. The theory behind low-cabohydrate diets is that when the body does not receive enough carbohydrate to function it starts to burn glycogen, or stored fat. This process releases water which results in immediate weight loss. In the long term, willfully to deprive the body of what it needs and replace it with foods that are higher in fat and lower in nutrients is doomed to failure. Some diets are particularly dangerous as they limit intake not only of grains but also most pulses, fruits and vegetables, thus depriving the dieter of fibre, vitamins and anti-oxidants.

I recall one Chinese cooking class where a lovely student asked me if she could leave the strips of carrot out of the Black Pepper Beef because her husband was on a diet called 'fat-busters' which had zero tolerance of carbohydrate. She, on the other hand, was on a high-fibre diet and had brought her own supply of brown rice. I didn't see how their kitchen could be much of a scene of unity and togetherness.

Along with some wonderful and interesting women, practically every type of food fanatic passed through the door of my cooking school. Each seemed to take ownership of his or her favourite diet plan and seemed completely confident that, based on the latest research, it was the only way to keep off the pounds. Sometimes they sounded so convincing that I wondered if perhaps I was wrong; but then I remembered that my argument, which is not a diet plan but a style of eating that is a way of life, has more than 3,000 years of Chinese history behind it and more than a billion slim people on its side.

At the end of each cooking class my helpers and I would lay the table with a colourful array of food which seldom failed to raise cries of admiration, along with the usual comments, 'We'll never get through all this,' and 'I won't need to eat tonight.' I always hoped there might be leftovers and then I wouldn't have to cook myself. Generally, though, all the dishes were finished, with the rich spicy deep-fried ones going first — only the rice would be left untouched. While my clients expounded their views on diet and weight loss I would often slip to the kitchen for an extra helping of rice and find Xiao Ding and her assistant, Xiao Niu, happily eating their staple from large rice bowls, twice the size of the decorative ones we used in the school.

Rice

If we are to embrace rice in our western kitchens we have to become familiar with its different varieties and learn how to cook it. In recent years not only health food shops, but supermarkets, too, have begun to stock an impressive range of rice varieties. The most common types are *indica* (long grain) and *japonica* (short grain). In China polished white rice has been favoured over brown out of necessity: whole grains are difficult to transport and store because vermin know a good thing when they find it. I learnt to love the Beijing short grain rice, but have been thrilled to see how in the health conscious West of the new millennium we at last have access to the true building blocks of a healthy diet. My new favourite is the short whole grain rice that has all the stickiness of the rice I enjoyed in Beijing but with extra nuttiness and nutrition too. Red rice from the Camargue makes an interesting change and can be mixed with other long grain or Basmati varieties. Experiment and find whichever type of rice you and your family enjoy, but try to avoid the over-processed 'easy cook' varieties. Wild rice (which isn't actually rice at all) adds flavour and texture when mixed with plain white or brown wholegrain rice. Then there is the black rice from southern China which leeches colour so is best served on its own (the Chinese usually use it only for porridge) when you want a colour contrast in your meal.

Most grains come complete with cooking instructions, but if you learn to work without needing to consult them, meal preparation will be less stressful. Rice is not difficult to cook in a saucepan by the 'thumbnail' method. Put in the rice and add water until it reaches the height of the joint on your thumb when the end of the nail (clipped short of course) is touching the rice. Cover and bring to the boil, then simmer until all the water is absorbed. Or, even better, buy a rice cooker, then you can always have cooked rice on hand and freeze the leftovers. Thawed rice is fantastic for frying and fried rice is one of the quickest and easiest meals to prepare.

When Xiao Ding visited the UK ten years ago the choice of grains on the market was much more limited than it is today – and in any case, she missed her particular variety of China's favourite staple. The Beijing rice is short grain, slightly sticky and tremendously satisfying. She thought our easy-cook varieties were tasteless by comparison, and Basmati was too fragrant for her liking. I sympathized and spent a fortune buying the short grain Japanese rice that was the best imitation, if slightly too stodgy. The following year Xiao Ding accompanied us to the UK a second time. She met us at the airport, dragging my favourite suitcase behind her. I knew better than to say anything, as there is a fine line between borrowing and taking, but I was surprised that she had needed to 'borrow' such a large piece of luggage. On her first trip she had packed an extensive wardrobe, appearing at breakfast in a pink and yellow flowered two-piece with a miniskirt; though when she found the rest of us in jeans or tracksuits she reserved her best clothes for photo opportunities. My hopes that the case might be half empty were dashed when I took hold of the handle to swing it on to the trolley and found I could barely lift it. 'What on earth have you got in

Simple fried rice
Chao fan

炒饭

Boiled rice is the more usual accompaniment to *cai*, though elaborate versions of fried rice feature in banquets. This simple recipe is generally made to use up leftovers. We often eat it for breakfast.

If you don't have any leftovers you will achieve a better result by cooking the rice the day before, leaving it in the fridge overnight then breaking it up roughly before using.

500 g/1 lb/2 cups leftover cooked rice
(brown, white or a mixture)
2 eggs, beaten
1 slice of ham optional, chopped into small squares
1 spring onion, finely chopped
50 g/2 oz/½ cup cooked peas
½ tsp salt (or to taste)
1 tbsp oil

Heat the wok to a high heat, add half the oil, and let it heat up. Tip in the beaten egg, allow it to puff up then stir it as it cooks to break it up. Remove the egg with a slotted spoon and set aside, allowing the excess oil to sink to the base of the wok.

Add the remainder of the oil, then the spring onion and the rice, and stir with a spatula until all the grains are separated. Turn the heat down slightly if the mixture is browning. Add the chopped ham, egg and peas and stir them in well.

Season with salt, mix well and serve.

there?' I gasped, wondering how we would manage the baggage allowance. She looked at me as if I was stupid: 'Rice,' she answered.

Or any other grain . . .

Because the Chinese diet has such an infinite variety of *cai*, (dishes), Chinese diners often enjoy their *fan*, or staple, plainly cooked and, as I learned from Xiao Ding, they tend to become very attached to their local type of rice. She once explained to me that rice was still a novelty to many Beijingers because before 1941 the area did not have irrigation systems to grow rice as staple crop, so the diet was based on wheat. Certainly Beijing is famous for the dumplings and flat-breads I have already mentioned, and also noodles and pancakes. Compared with rice though, these are generally regarded as lighter options, to be eaten when time is short.

For modern living, combination dishes such as fried noodles, offering both *fan* and *cai*, have the advantage of convenience, and while I came to love rice and seldom go a day without using it in at least one meal, I like to use different grains or pasta and often mix my vegetables in with them, fusion style. New varieties of staple foods are reaching western supermarket shelves all the time. Barley is ideal for risottos; the protein-packed quinoa makes a tasty salad, cornmeal (polenta) and water makes a pizza-type base, and the soaked and steamed grain is delicious cut in slices and fried.

Bread

So what's wrong with sandwiches anyway? For many of us in the West, bread is such an integral part of our diet that the thought of giving it up overnight is terrifying (though many people have had to because of the rise in gluten allergies). If you like bread, and it likes you, then you can still enjoy our western favourite as a staple food. Better and more interesting varieties of bread are appearing in the West all the time, and there is no doubt that the stoneground, organic varieties featuring wholegrain 'designer' flours and even nuts and seeds, are superior nutritionally to the white, sliced equivalent. Enjoy fresh interesting breads with your meals, but with moderation. Much of the bread we eat is processed and packed with preservatives.

Fan, staples to eat away from home

- curried brown-rice salad with blanched beansprouts, peanuts, raisins and honey-mustard dressing
- pasta salad with tuna, sweetcorn, tomato, olives and anchovies
- buckwheat noodles with sweet potato, marinated bean-curd, shredded spring onions and soy sauce
- couscous with stir-fried red and yellow peppers, almonds and sultanas
- quinoa with minced ginger, chopped, blanched green beans, squares of tofu or ham, and sesame oil

Sandwich fillings are often primarily animal protein with a token vegetable garnish, and generally bread does not lend itself to partnering interesting vegetable dishes in the same way as a loose grain or a noodle-style product. In northern China people make fresh *mantou* (steamed buns) on a daily basis. Simple to make with either yeast or baking powder, *mantou* can be made with white or wholemeal flower or a mixture. They only take a few minutes to knead and can be steamed in twelve to fifteen minutes. *Mantou* are eaten alongside *cai* in place of, or sometimes as well as, rice. Sometimes they are spread with fermented beancurd 'cheese', a tasty savoury spread. Because they are made without preservatives and their eating quality is one of soft freshness, *mantou* are always eaten on the day they are steamed. The whole eating experience is very different from one where bread is treated as a convenience food and a piece of toast is seen as a substitute for a real meal. Freshly-made wholegrain bread is a great food, but don't rely on it too much and find yourself eating a limited diet.

If you are a habitual dieter, the the idea of basing your meals on grain foods may seem radical, but remember that Chinese people have based their diet on carbohydrates for thousands of years, and that plainly-boiled staples, especially wholegrain ones, are low in fat and high in nutrients and fibre. Staple foods are cheap, easy to prepare, incredibly versatile and delicious and satisfying to eat, especially when accompanied by freshly cooked *cai* (vegetable dishes).

Steamed bread
Mantou

These simple buns are a popular staple food in northern China, often eaten with *cai* instead of rice. They are also good with soup or *zhou*, or simply on their own. Chinese people spread them with fermented red beancurd cheese, but butter is an option.

Mantou are simple (and sociable) to make but there are several stages to the recipe, so a little forward planning is needed. *Mantou* are best eaten freshly steamed, but, in the unlikely event that you have any left over, they will keep 48 hours in a tin.

This recipe can be made either with white or wholemeal flour, but a 60–40 mix of white to wholemeal works best. Depending on the size of *mantou* you require, this recipe will make 16–24. Bigger *mantou* (some are as big as a tennis ball) tend to be moister and keep longer.

25 g/¾ oz/⅛ cup dried yeast
½ tsp salt
2 tbsp sugar
500 ml/16 fl oz/2 cups warm water
800 g/1lb 11 oz/8 cups flour
2 tbsp oil

Put the yeast, salt and sugar in a bowl. Add a small amount of the water, dissolve the yeast, then add the rest of the water. Leave to stand in a warm place for 15 minutes or until frothy.

Sieve the flour into a large mixing bowl; make a well in the centre and pour in the liquid, gradually working in the dough. When all the water is incorporated, continue to work the dough for a few minutes until soft and smooth and all the flour from the edges of the basin has been incorporated. Add the oil and work it in.

Cover the bowl with a damp cloth and leave in a very warm place for 1 ½ hours. The dough should double in size.

Pick up the dough and divide it into two. It will be quite sticky and you may need to flour your hands. Divide each half of the dough into 8–12 pieces.

Taking one small piece of dough at a time, place it on the palm of one hand to form a small ball. Flatten it slightly so that you have a little round cushion and use the other to pull the outside edges in to the centre. Then turn it over and flatten it on a level surface to make a flat roundish piece. Roll this into a rough sausage shape, then pick it up and roll it between your palms. Then, using this new ball, repeat the process a few times to work the dough. Finish each piece by rolling it between your palms so you have a small ball. Place each ball on a piece of greaseproof paper, flattening the base slightly and move on to the next piece of dough.

When all the *mantou* are ready place them in a steaming basket and leave in a very warm place for half an hour to allow the dough to rise again.

Finally, steam for 12–15 minutes and eat as soon as possible.

four

Eat until you are full

四

'Whilst travelling don't reckon the distance; whilst eating
don't reckon the quantity.'

OLD CHINESE PROVERB

The Chinese eat until they are full – and then they stop. A
phrase that is uttered almost as often as 'Have you eaten yet?'
is '*Wo chi bao le*' ('I've eaten until I'm full'). The statement is
not questioned because it doesn't need to be. 'Full' doesn't
mean 'Oh, I would love some more but I won't because I am
watching my weight.' It means full.

Sounds great, doesn't it? Filling up on western food is not
difficult either, especially now that our diet has become so
international. Breakfast could be eggs, bacon, sausage, tomato,
mushrooms and fried bread, or croissants and pastries. If we
were not counting our calories we might well enjoy a pizza
at lunch-time, followed by our favourite ice-cream, and stop
for tea or coffee with cakes or biscuits in the middle of the
afternoon. And for those with the time to cook or the opportunity to eat out, a gourmet meal might include a deep-fried

starter, a main fish or meat course with a rich, creamy sauce and chips on the side, followed by a gooey pudding and cheese. But eating like this doesn't always result in a sensation of satisfaction – more often in an uncomfortable, bloated feeling, a surreptitious undoing of the waistband and a wash of guilt as we reach for a chocolate to eat with our coffee. Whether or not we count calories we know that we can't eat this way every day without risking weight gain, or worse. This is why we now we have the 'healthy options': muesli and yoghurt in place of the fry-up, a Caesar or Niçoise salad lunch (with low-fat dressing). Sadly though, low-fat, low-calorie meals tend to be distinctly uninteresting: scour a restaurant menu and you might find a slice of melon, a house salad, grilled chicken breast or salmon steak and a range of fruit sorbets. Faced with these rather bland and dry options, many people prefer a pattern of indulgence and denial.

I was once asked by a major retailer to put together an itinerary for a group of food technicians to help them deepen their understanding of authentic northern Chinese food. I took them to the countryside where we feasted on freshly-picked soya beans boiled until tender with Sichuan peppercorns and star anise, smashed cucumber with garlic and chilli and little cornmeal cakes topped with lightly scrambled egg and bright green Chinese chives. But they didn't really pay attention until I demonstrated a lamb stir-fry. Are the English too conservative for soya beans or are the margins much better on lamb, I wondered.

Enjoying sumptuous evening meals and lots of wine in Beijing's top restaurants, my clients outlined the eating habits of the typical British consumer. People who want to 'be good', the euphemism for losing weight, or eat what they regard as a healthy options, do so from Monday to Friday, the marketing director confided. Many people starve themselves all week so that from Friday night to Monday morning they can have maximum taste and satisfaction. 'This is what the ready-meals market tries to offer,' he said. 'So we've got to forget the tofu and vegetables and think about rich meals made of meat.'

Wouldn't it be better, I tried to suggest, to eat tasty and satisfying meals every day of the week? Could they not promote a diet that would make nutritious food a way of life instead of an optional extra? No one took me seriously; for a start they didn't believe such a phenomenon was possible and in any case their target was only two to three meals per week per household.

Multi-dish eating

The Chinese diet doesn't countenance overindulgence, but it doesn't have 'healthy options' either. People eat well at every meal, never making do with a couple of snacks and one main eating occasion. One great advantage of the Chinese style of eating is its multi-dish approach. Chinese meals do not have a centrepiece: the dishes arrive on the table in random order so that everyone can take a little from each of a selection of different foods. The variety of foods relieves the diners from the burden of choice and their palates from boredom. It is a relaxed and stress-free way of eating, with everyone using chopsticks to select tasty morsels from the various dishes. A Chinese table always promises satisfaction yet it is almost impossible to count calories by the chopstick-full.

In China no single ingredient is ever served in large quantities; the preference is always for a large number of different foods served in manageable amounts. Rather than increase the quantity of any particular dish, a Chinese chef will add another element to a meal. Cold dishes and stir-fries are usually served on small dinner plates or in shallow soup or cereal bowls, which show off the chef's exquisite knife work, rather than in large, irregularly shaped containers which would hide their qualities from view. The table might also feature a simmering tray and a clay pot, and always a big a bowl of soup. By taking a little from each of the dishes the diner soon feels satiated. It is bad manners to take too much of any one dish and good manners to try a little of everything. This enables all the diners to consume a feast without feeling uncomfortable.

Children who are brought up to eat in this fashion are never overwhelmed by a mound of food. A child is much more likely to experiment with a small tasting of a new ingredient when everyone else is digging in and there is no pressure. In this way they learn to listen to their own appetites and so do not fall into the 'American portion' trap, where larger quantities promise more satisfaction, and which, when combined with a lifelong habit of 'clearing the plate', can lead to eating too much of the wrong things in adulthood. There is, incidentally, no concept of 'children's food' in Asia, although many of the colourful and interesting dishes appeal to a youngster's sense of adventure.

Eat promiscuously

In my journey into Chinese food culture I inevitably moved away from the type of Chinese dishes favoured by 'foreigners' towards those enjoyed by native Chinese people. Sometimes even I found myself outside of my comfort zone. Yet the more I ate, firstly in terms of quantity but most importantly in terms of variety, the better I felt. To really benefit from the Chinese approach you too need to be adventurous and accept that you cannot limit your diet to the foods you prefer.

The Chinese poet Huang Ting Jian, writing in the eleventh century, listed three bad attitudes: 'To be greedy for something palatable, to shun what is unpalatable and to be oblivious to the source of what one eats.' He could also have said: 'Don't be fussy and squeamish, or always choose what is tasty and convenient.' Either way his voice would most likely have fallen on deaf ears in today's society.

Our dietary preferences are strongly defined by cultural boundaries that we are all too often blissfully unaware of, especially as 'foreign foods' in our own countries are cleverly adapted to local tastes so as to give us the illusion that we are cosmo politan in our eating habits. The nature of the western diet does not encourage promiscuous eating, instead it forces people to chose one main ingredient per meal, be it a cut of meat, a topping for pizza or pasta or a sandwich filling, and this leads people into the habit of eating the same foods over and over again, foods that are not necessarily providing total satisfaction or sufficient nourishment.

After a few years in China I became completely at ease with fungus and beancurd in its many varieties, and was not averse to seaweed, but I still found that while the students on my cooking course genuinely wanted to learn about Chinese food, they were very conservative about what they were prepared to eat. We would take a trip through the market and pass through a tempting array of street stalls, where I would buy a few of the green eggs that my children, as Dr Seuss fans, considered to be a natural partner to ham. After three months in quicklime, the yolk of these eggs turns black while the white becomes a transparent, greenish jelly. The objective of the process, which I imagine was discovered by accident, is to achieve a new combination of textures. The yolk becomes creamy and the white transforms to something akin to gelatine. At lunch-time we would peel and quarter the eggs and dress them with a simple mixture of minced ginger, soy sauce and sesame oil. My advice was always to close your eyes and take a bite. Those who had the courage to try were pleasantly surprised.

The Chinese know when to stop eating since they are relaxed in the knowledge that the next meal will be as good and filling as the one they are savouring at the time. And the nature of Chinese food is such that they have time to savour it because they use chopsticks to select small pieces from the array of dishes in front of them. With less food per bite, but more bites overall, the meal is both physiologically and psychologically satisfying. When the stomach is given enough time to realize that it is full, and the mind has time to recognize this feeling, the overall sensation of satiety is very different from the one of physical engorgement that we often associate with being full in the West.

Learning to eat Chinese style

In my early days in China I used to watch Xiao Ding arrive every day with a steel container. These, I soon learnt, are used all over China to keep food warm away from home. The smell of her meal would always make me realize how hungry I was, whether or not I had eaten my own lunch. I was desperate to exchange my sandwich and salad for a feast like hers, but a mixture of shyness and uneasiness in our relationship prevented me from enquiring about the contents of her lunch-box, which appeared to provide a meal that was so much more satisfying and filling than the food I was accustomed to.

One day I sat with my mouth-watering as she devoured a pile of little dumplings, each one oozing fragrant juices, and decided that I had to pluck up the courage to ask her to teach me to make some. She was reluctant at first, telling me that because our two food cultures were so markedly different, I would never be able to enjoy Chinese food on a regular basis. But when she eventually relented we had a riot – and I found the first of many uses for the enormous Beijing cabbages that are piled up all over town throughout the winter.

Jiaozi – *boiled dumplings*

Chinese families get together on the eve of Chinese New Year and make little dumplings called *jiaozi*. Both the act of making them and the shape and form of the dumplings symbolize unity, the new moon and the idea that everything goes full circle. Perhaps Xiao Ding thought about all this when we started our culinary journey together, or perhaps someone had told her that all foreigners like dumplings. For me, at least, it was a symbolic moment and *jiaozi* remain our favourite family dish.

Jiaozi have an infinite variety of fillings, usually encompassing a small amount of meat but often vegetarian too, and like everything else in China they are consumed in massive bowlfuls. With the assurance that Chinese people have when explaining anything food-related, Xiao Ding told me that the average man would eat half a *jin*, about one pound, at a sitting, which is around twenty-five dumplings. It is usual, Xiao Ding told me confidently, for women to eat *san liang* or three-tenths

Boiled dumplings
Jiaozi

饺子

Ingredients for about 30 jiaozi:
250 g/8 oz/2 cups plain flour
(high-gluten if possible – a mixture of half
wholemeal and half unbleached white works well)
150 ml/5 fl oz/¾ cup cold water
(a little more if you use wholemeal flour)
a pinch of salt

For the filling:
150 g/5½ oz/¾ cup outdoor bred porkk mince
1 tsp cooking wine
1 tsp finely chopped ginger
1 tsp finely chopped spring onion
100g/3½ oz/1 cup vegetables such as Chinese cabbage,
dill, carrot, green beans or Chinese chives
1 tsp sesame oil
1 tsp Chinese cooking wine
1 tsp soy sauce
salt to taste

Gradually add the water to the flour, mixing into a stiff dough. Knead for a few minutes and roll into a ball. Cover with a damp tea-towel and leave to rest while you make the filling.

Chop the vegetable very finely. Note that some vegetables require pre-treatment as follows:

White cabbage: sprinkle with salt, wrap in a towel and squeeze out excess liquid.

Beans and carrots: blanch for three to five minutes (longer for beans), then squeeze out excess water.

Put the meat in the bowl, add the seasonings, finely-chopped spring onion and ginger and, lastly, the finely-chopped vegetable.

Flour a flat surface, then take half the lump of dough, roll it into a sausage about 2½cm (1in) in diameter. Break off a small ball, then, using a rolling-pin, roll it out into a circle with the edges thinner than the middle. Take the circle onto the palm of your hand, and place a small amount (about 1tsp) of the filling in the centre. Fold into a little crescent-shaped purse, by first pulling two opposite sides together, then pinching and pleating each side. Arrange the dumplings on the tray, making sure that they do not touch each other.

When you are ready to cook the *jiaozi*, bring a large pan of water to the boil. Add the *jiaozi*, taking care not to break them up or to overfill the pan. Stir very gently to ensure they do not stick to the bottom and bring the water back to the boil: do not let it boil too vigorously.

There are several methods of cooking *jiaozi*. The best one for beginners is to add a small cup of cold water each time the water comes to the boil. When you have added three cups the *jiaozi* will be cooked, and because the water has not been allowed to boil rapidly the skins will not be broken. Cooked *jiaozi* float to the top and have wrinkly puckered skins. If in doubt, test one! Remove with a slotted spoon.

Tomato and egg filling

A simple vegetarian filling can be made from tomato and egg.

4 tomatoes

3 eggs

2tsp oil

½tsp finely-chopped ginger
½tsp finely-chopped spring onion
½tsp salt
2tsp sesame oil

Blanch the tomatoes and remove the skins. Cut in half, take out the seeds and squeeze out the excess liquid, then chop roughly.

Beat the eggs. Heat the wok to a high heat, add oil and tip in the eggs. Allow them to fluff up, then stir so that they break into tiny pieces. Turn off the heat then add the ginger and spring onion and season with a little salt and sesame oil.

Make *jiaozi* in exactly the same way as for the meat recipe; this filling is a little more difficult to handle so be careful it does not 'leak' into the edges of the dumplings, since this will cause them to break up during cooking.

Jiaozi with this filling take very little time to cook. Add them to the boiling water as directed above, bring back to the boil and they should be ready. Test one! *Jiaozi* are served without a sauce, but with simple accompaniments such as rich black vinegar and chilli oil for dipping.

of a *jin*, and, right on cue, I packed away fifteen before announcing that I had *chi bao le* – eaten 'till I was full'.

Xiao Ding and I shared many a lunch at the kitchen table. We ate a lot of noodles, in soup or with tasty sauces made from minced beef and green beans, aubergine and tomato or, on adventurous days, dried mushrooms with wood-ear fungus.

Sometimes we would make dumplings, boiled or steamed, or *wontons* in soup, but we both loved rice-based meals the most. In a working day we ate a mound of one of the common favourites: spicy cabbage, potato slices with green chilli, shredded daikon radish and carrot with cumin, tender chunks of tofu with Sichuan peppercorns. Sometimes we would make a couple of side dishes: mashed cucumber with chilli and garlic, boiled quail's eggs with five-spice, or a bowl of steaming soup. In the winter we often feasted on a lamb and radish or a chicken and vegetable stew. Whenever I cooked with Xiao Ding she appeared to know exactly what quantity to prepare so that we would clear the plates feeling distinctly satisfied yet not uncomfortable. To encourage the weighing and measuring of ingredients would not be in the spirit of the Chinese way. It took me a long time to acquire Xiao Ding's innate ability to judge portion size. But, spurred on by her slim figure and clear complexion, I gradually began to increase my portions until I always finished my meal feeling that I had eaten just the right amount.

At this moment you may be thinking, 'That's all very well, but I don't have time to make dumplings, I can't afford quail's eggs and there is no way I'm eating wood-ear fungus.' Or you may be wondering instead if it is acceptable to eat chips and cheeseburgers, chocolate cake or Häagen-Daz until you are full.

It is common knowledge that eating more fast food or sugar-laden snacks is not the way forward on the path to a slim, fit and healthy body. This book is about introducing you to a lifestyle that will satisfy your body to an extent that daily battles with the fat and sugar-loaded 'baddies' of the western diet will cease to become an issue.

I haven't made dumplings for months and, now that I live in the UK, wood-ear fungus is just an occasional treat. I hope that you will try these delicacies at some time, but there are also ways of preparing satisfying meals without having to grapple with unfamiliar ingredients or follow complicated recipes. I will help you to do so as I unveil further secrets; but for now just think about adding more variety to your diet as you adopt a multi-dish way of eating and try to listen to your body's response.

This approach can be daunting: just remember that the general Chinese rule is one dish per person, with rice, and that dishes can be as simple as a plate of sliced tomatoes with a sprinkling of minced spring onion, salt, sugar and sesame oil, or blanched green beans topped with minced ginger, sesame oil and soy sauce.

Here, for instance, is an example of a Chinese-influenced lunch that I recently prepared in the UK for a group of Tim's Chinese business colleagues. All the foods were available from my local supermarket and the simple dishes featured just one or two main ingredients and took less than ten minutes each to prepare.

To start, I served cold mixed celery with boiled peanuts. This was followed by stir-fried courgettes with cumin and chilli, tomatoes with egg, spicy cabbage with tofu, broccoli with garlic, a beef and potato stew and a large steamed salmon topped with shredded ginger and spring onion. Everyone ate a large bowl of rice or two, and finally I served a soup. There were eight of us in total and we cleared the plates. As a token English gesture I had made an apple crumble to finish. A couple of guests opted to sample a small portion, but most declined, saying that they were full or that they didn't particularly like sweet foods. I didn't persevere, knowing that when Chinese people say they have '*chi bao le*' they mean it, and it's a compliment. I thought momentarily of my friend in the London restaurant, playing with her food to save her calories for the

If you reach for a Chinese recipe book and try to make multi-dish meals from scratch you may well be overwhelmed. Better, perhaps, to start off with meals you are already familiar with.

For example, if you have a family of four and plan to eat Chilli-con-carne with French bread and green salad, make a bowl of chilli, stir-fry some mushrooms (perhaps add some baby spinach leaves), slice some tomatoes and cucumber and chop and roast a butternut squash, topped with crushed garlic and herbs and drizzled with olive oil. Put all the dishes in the centre of the table, give everyone a bowl of rice and let them dig in.

Or, instead of grilled chicken breasts, try a chicken stir-fry accompanied with stewed red and yellow peppers and beansprouts; open a tin of kidney beans and stew them with tomatoes and spices, mash or slice an avocado or two, grate some cheese and serve with tortillas or pancakes.

Even a simple supper of baked potatoes can be made into a multi-course meal. Most of the dishes suggested above make good toppings; alternatively, try curried prawns, cauliflower with cheese, or a spiced vegetable mix with coconut.

肉　蔬菜

chocolate mousse and *petit fours*, and wondered if she ever felt truly satisfied after a meal.

Chinese people know when they have had enough, but that is because they have had enough; the Chinese have a positive relationship with eating and are in control of their appetites, but they also eat substantial amounts of good food. My journey into Chinese food culture has led me to believe that denial or restriction of a person's natural appetite will never solve the West's burgeoning obesity problem and health-related issues. A person who is constantly hungry will never fit comfortably into his or her body. If the Chinese can *chi bao le* at every meal without getting fat, then so can you.

The basics

The first four secrets of the Chinese diet come together into a common-sense eating plan: enjoy your eating, base your meals around vegetables, accompanied by a generous portion of a staple food, and eat as much as your appetite dictates. Before you know it you will find that you are forgetting to count calories.

'But that's too simple!' you cry – and perhaps a little boring? 'There must be more to the Chinese food culture than vegetables and rice?' You are right: read on . . .

吃饱了

In order to *chi bao le*, try to incorporate these principles into the way you eat:

- Have the confidence to eat well and regularly. If you do, you won't get so hungry that you don't have the willpower to prepare a meal so snack on empty calories instead.
- If eating larger meals makes you feel bloated and uncomfortable, it could be your body adjusting to a healthier regime. Or you could be sensitive to some foods; listen to your body, it will tell you what suits it if you just give it time.
- Use the multi-dish approach. Place the food in the centre of the table and place small amounts onto your plate.
- Savour each mouthful. The multi-dish approach allows you to think about what you are eating, rather than clearing a plate without even noticing.
- Don't eat too quickly. Remember that your appetite takes a while to register how much you have eaten. Experiment with chopsticks. They will help you be more aware of what you are eating and slow you down too.

five

Take liquid food

五

'As long as there is rice, there should be soup.'

LI YU (1611–80)

Cai and *fan*, dishes and staples, should now be completely within your grasp; but lurking behind them are two other categories of food. The rich and flavoursome *cai* has its partner in the light and often insipid watery soup known as *tang*. *Fan*, which encompasses cooked rice, noodles and all manner of delicious breads and pancakes, has a liquid equivalent called *zhou*, consumed by the gallon all over the China, particularly first thing in the morning. Made by simmering rice in about ten times its volume of water, *zhou* is sometimes known in the West by its southern Chinese name, *congee*. 'Porridge' is a common, though rather a florid, translation though 'gruel' is more accurate.

No Chinese meal is complete without a bowl of soup, but *tang* rarely resembles its western counterpart. The south of China is famous for its rich but delicate consommé-type preparations, served towards the beginning of the meal, as in the West. But in the north a water-based broth is usually served after the rice, in the same bowl so as to ensure that not a single grain of the precious *fan* is wasted. More of a drink than something to eat, these Chinese soups could be mistaken for the water left after washing up the saucepan.

If you have taken on board the ideas expressed in the preceding chapters you will be eating more vegetable-based *cai*, experimenting with new ingredients and increasing the variety in your diet. Your whole food experience will be enhanced, whether you are eating in Chinese style or adapting your western cooking. Adopting the Chinese approach to *fan* and eating more and different staple foods may have been an effort at first, especially as there are so many prejudices about starchy foods, but it will have simply involved a change of emphasis rather than a totally new food experience.

As we move on to the fifth secret of the Chinese diet, and I introduce the concepts of *tang* (soup), and *zhou* (porridge), you may have to move out of your comfort zone in pursuit of a new relationship with food. My teaching experience showed me that if there were any leftover dishes after a meal it would be the stews, braises and soups. Western appetites, I have seen, show a strong preference for rich foods over light ones, solid textures over soft and dry over liquid dishes.

As our western diet is generally too dry, some of the worst offenders are the 'healthy' products like rice cakes, oatcakes, cereal bars and toasted muesli. The need to drink water seems to have increased in direct proportion with the denaturing of our diet. In recent years western nutritionists have been urging us to drink more water, providing yet another opportunity for food and drink manufacturers to foist hoards of new designer brands on us all. Drinking water with meals may have a negative effect on digestion and absorption and drinking copious amounts of water through the day does not necessarily benefit health, as Jill Fullerton–Smith showed in the BBC TV series *The Truth about Food*. In China you seldom see anyone drink water while they are eating. While Chinese restaurants have begun to offer a range of soft drinks, presumably because they are good earners, traditionally taking a drink with food has been considered damaging to the stomach. Instead, every meal contains a liquid element, and of course the vegetable bias of the meals ensures a high water content.

Yin *and* yang

I have met very few westerners who like *tang* or *zhou*, Chinese soups or porridge on first tasting. So why should we include them in our diet? Isn't Chinese cooking all about making ingredients taste good? Generally this is true, but it is also about achieving balance and harmony.

Now it is time to introduce the Taoist concept of *yin* and *yang*, which pervades every area of Chinese thought and life: every mountain has a sunny and a shady side; one cannot exist without the other and because they contain a small amount of the other's nature, so they can transform each other. Nothing, therefore, is either all good, or all bad.

Gone are the days when we were told to 'Eat up, it's good for you.' Perhaps the Great Tao can help us understand where our parents and teachers have failed. *Yin* and *yang* are not so much opposites as potential. From the dark and passive female *yin*, the bright and active male *yang* is born. This might be a difficult concept for the western mind, trained to think of a square as a square and not as a would-be circle; but, once grasped, this idea opens up a world of possibilities. A *like* becomes a potential *dislike* and a *dislike* a potential *like*. When *yin* and *yang* is applied to the Chinese diet, *zhou* and *tang* can be better understood. *Fan*, or rice, is potential *zhou*; in fact I often make *zhou* from leftover rice. *Cai* is a potential *tang*, with many combinations, tomato and egg for example, used both in dishes and soups.

Tang – *soup*

Like everything else in Chinese cooking, soup makes sense from a nutritional but also an environmental point of view. My grandfather used to make my mother drink the water he had used to cook the vegetables. This was standing joke in our family until the time we rented a courtyard house in a small peasant village just outside Beijing and found that the water supply was restricted. Though the owner had warned us to take bottles, of course we forgot, and then were horrified to find that our limited supply had run out. Suddenly my children were faced with the option of either going thirsty or of drinking the water which I had used to blanch the broccoli. Chinese soups are slightly more interesting than tepid broccoli water, but the concept is often the same. They usually combine two or more complementary or contrasting ingredients and a couple of chunks of ginger and spring onion to flavour the stock. Leafy greens feature heavily and other ingredients might include egg, meat or offal, fish, seafood, dried mushrooms or other fungus, seaweed or tofu. Sesame oil or chopped coriander is often sprinkled on the top to add fragrance, and white pepper is used to add a kick and to help digestion.

Because most people do not adopt the Taoist approach to eating, I have made a real effort over the years to find some

Chinese soups that are to the western taste. I used to include three simple recipes in my classes. My favourite was a light vegetable recipe with a mixture of textures, but I found that most of my students felt indifferently about it. There was an unusual combination of winter melon, which is a bit like a marrow but with a smoother texture, and pork balls, which my children loved. Then Xiao Ding introduced me to a delicate white combination of grated Chinese (daikon) radish and cellophane noodles topped with crisply fried Sichuan peppercorns.

The fluid element in your diet doesn't have to be the washing up water type, either; any type of liquid food is nourishing. This is one area where many food cultures have something to offer. Minestrone, Scotch broth, mulligatawny and various chowders are all packed with nutrients. Practically every leafy or root vegetable can be made into soup, and pulses are a convenient and nutritious addition. Traditional combinations include pea and lettuce, leek and potato and curried parsnip. I like to add Asian flavours to my soups: pumpkin or butternut squash with ginger and red chilli, finished with a splash of coconut milk; red or brown lentils with cumin, coriander, garlic and fresh green chilli. Invest in a handheld blender and you can make all manner of thick soups, and thus find yet another way to increase the range of vegetables in your diet.

One way to make a light and nutritious broth is to boil, rather than fry, all the ingredients, including the supporting vegetables such as onion, garlic or chilli, and then add a splash of a good-quality cold pressed oil just before serving. Depending on the flavour required, any combination of whole cloves of garlic, pieces of ginger and spring onion, shallots, pieces of dried red chilli or other herbs and spices may be added to the water. The garlic cloves and onion pieces can be peeled and then blended with the main ingredients, although other additions are best removed with a slotted spoon to avoid crunchy bits in the finished soup.

Zhou – *porridge*

So much for soup. *Zhou,* or porridge, is something else again. I have now eaten it for breakfast every day for the past two years and quite often as a snack, so if I don't have it, I miss it terribly. But when my nine-year-old son put it on his list of 'hates' for a school assignment, along with jellied eggs – a lightly steamed concoction that is Xiao Ding's favourite cure for diarrhoea – I had a degree of sympathy. There is nothing visually inviting about a bowl of white slop and the whole eating experience is very different from what we are accustomed to in the West.

I first tasted *zhou* when we were in the countryside up by the Miyun reservoir, under the shadow of one of the tributaries of the Great Wall. We stayed in a traditional courtyard house, devoid of plumbing or central heating, which belonged to the charismatic Guo Gui Lan, a forceful fifty-something country woman. Millet porridge was standard early-morning fare, topped with a fried egg if you were a paying customer, and we all knew better than to ask Guo Gui Lan for an alternative. Unlike rice *zhou*, which is quite slimy and very light in taste, millet porridge has a slightly nutty flavour and grainy texture. In western terms, millet is full of vitamins and rich in iron, so there are plenty of reasons for persevering with it.

More common, however, is *mi zhou* or rice porridge. The short, slightly sticky Beijing rice lends itself well to boiling for several hours in about ten times its volume in water, until

White radish soup
Luo bo tang

萝卜汤

Although it can be eaten raw, this vegetable (also known as daikon or mooli) is most commonly used in stews, with lamb or pork, and soups. This simple recipe is for a light, cleansing soup, which goes well with richer dishes. You can add pork balls for a more substantial dish.

1 medium white daikon radish (mooli),
shredded or grated
1 litre/2 pints/5 cups water
a few slices of ginger
a few slices of spring onion
100 g/3½ oz/1 cup cellophane (mung-bean) noodles
2 tsp oil
1 tsp Sichuan peppercorns
2 tsp sesame oil
1 bunch of coriander, roughly chopped
½ tsp salt or to taste
1 tsp white pepper or to taste

Bring the water to the boil in a saucepan. Add ginger, spring onion and radish and simmer for three minutes without covering the pan. Add the cellophane noodles, and continue simmering for a further three minutes or until they are soft.

Heat the oil in the wok until very hot. Add the Sichuan peppercorns and allow them to sizzle until all the fragrance has been extracted (they should be nearly black). Tip the oil with peppercorns over the soup (sieving out the peppercorns if you do not want little black bits in your soup). Finally add the salt, a teaspoon or two of sesame oil and some white pepper and chopped coriander to garnish.

it forms a sloppy porridge. Whenever Xiao Ding made *baozi* (steamed dumplings) for lunch, she would make herself a bowl of *zhou* to eat alongside it. I am a great fan of the light bready buns stuffed with pork and cabbage seasoned with ginger and spring onion and I was always happy to share them with her. But when she offered me *zhou* as well, I never accepted, as it seemed like extra carbohydrate for no reason. Of course, I should have realized that there *was* a reason, obvious to anyone who understands the duality of *yin* and *yang*. 'The two foods', she explained, 'go together because dumplings are dry and porridge is wet.' From that day as I strolled the streets, I noticed how all Chinese people slurp *zhou* alongside their dumplings. The substance that is slopped out of steaming vats into cracked porcelain, or more recently, polystyrene bowls is more like porridge than gruel and it is consumed in volumes.

Once I had taken on board the whole concept of liquid food, I saw *zhou* everywhere. Not only is it served in all roadside stalls but it's also on every Chinese restaurant menu. In fact, there are whole restaurants devoted just to serving *zhou*. I found sweet *zhou* and savoury *zhou*; *zhou* with nuts, *zhou* with fruits, *zhou* with pulses, *zhou* with a range of meats and fish and *zhou* with every Chinese vegetable I knew and some that I didn't.

Rice *zhou* is the most common, but it can be made with millet, sorghum, buckwheat, corn and even a treasured grain called 'Job's tears' (coix seed) which looks a bit like pearl barley. Then there is the famous *ba bao zhou* ('eight treasure porridge') that is traditionally eaten on *La Ba*, the eighth day of the twelfth month, which heralds the onset of winter. The 'eight treasures' comprise a mixture of pulses, fruits and seeds that can vary from recipe to recipe. The concept is not so different from muesli, only whereas muesli can be heavy and difficult to digest, and both oats and wheat can cause problems in our allergy-prone modern society, *zhou* is lighter and based on rice, which is non-allergenic.

Getting rid of toxins

In China, nobody questions the many benefits of *zhou*. As well as being the perfect food for invalids – even those with a fever who in the West might not be given solid food – it is believed to have a cleansing effect, getting rid of toxins while preventing the body from dehydration. Anyone who has eaten at a real Chinese banquet or a celebratory meal in a good restaurant will know that the Chinese enjoy rich food from time to time and never talk about cutting back the next day. But they do eat *zhou*, to remedy the effect of serious overindulgence.

You may be wondering why a bowl of mushy rice should be better than, say, a blueberry smoothie or a glass of freshly-pressed vegetable juice, both bursting with vitamins to revitalize your system. Sometimes our digestive systems need a rest. One solution would be just to go hungry, but that in itself brings stresses and strains. Just as the best way into an exercise regime is through a gentle warm up, the digestive system needs to be started slowly after a night's rest or a period of sickness. The Chinese expression *kai wei'r* means literally 'to open the stomach', and this is exactly what *zhou* can do. My grandfather, though not familiar with *zhou* as such, would have agreed with the Chinese that a weak or tired body is best nourished by a steaming hot bowl of restorative broth.

It took me a long time to convert to the *zhou* habit, and I do not expect you to acquire it overnight. But if I can convince you to try it the benefits will probably make your efforts worthwhile. Before I started to eat *zhou* for breakfast I had accepted the fact that I suffered from headaches and a dry feeling in my mouth most mornings, and often felt bloated and uncomfortable. I knew from friends that these symptoms weren't uncommon and there were plenty of possible causes, ranging from the Beijing pollution to the impossibility of finding Sam's shoes on a school morning. I had even toyed with the newly fashionable idea that I suffered from wheat intolerance.

Since I have been eating *zhou* regularly these symptoms have practically disappeared, and I have not needed to sacrifice my former favourites. My appetite in the morning has increased and, when I have time, I eat steamed or freshly baked bread with my *zhou*, sometimes an egg as well. My newly balanced body does not react unfavourably if *zhou* is not an option and I eat a more conventional breakfast from time to time.

What is it about *zhou* that makes it so health-giving? The role of *zhou* becomes clearer if you understand that Chinese doctors apply the Taoist principles of *yin* and *yang* to the human body. A fit body has a perfect balance of these opposing forces. If a person is unwell, overtired or has simply over-indulged, Chinese people believe that the balance needs to be brought back into line.

Yin *and* yang *in the body*

According to Traditional Chinese Medicine, the inside of the body is *yin* and the surface is *yang*. *Yin* is everything that is passive and associated with storage; *yang* is active and responsible for processing. Our *Qi*, or life-force, is created from the perfect balance of *yin* and *yang*.

In Chinese dietary therapy, which is a branch of Traditional Chinese Medicine, foods are also classified as *yin* and *yang*. *Yin* foods move inwards and assist the functioning of the internal organs, while *yang* foods generally rise up and out towards the body surface, and can contribute to indigestion, skin problems and headaches if taken in excess. *Yang* foods usually have hot or warm energies and so create heat in the body, whereas *yin* foods usually have cold or cool properties and so cool the body down. It is possible, though, for foods to be *yang* (and move outwards), yet cooling (China's favourite fish, carp, is one example; another is peppermint) or even *yin* and warming (such as dried orange-peel).

Because a good Chinese diet is one that is balanced, it is important to avoid too much of one food property. Fortunately there are a number of neutral foods (both in terms of *yin* and *yang* and their hot or cold properties) that maintain the equilibrium in the body. Rice is neutral in terms of its heating and cooling properties, but very slightly *yang*. How a dish is cooked can affect its heating or cooling nature quite considerably, as we shall see. Generally though, wet and moist are *yin* characteristics of food, and dry and crisp are *yang*.

By taking rice, a neutral energy food that is slightly *yang*, and simmering it to create a moist end product, Chinese people create a food, *zhou,* that will not push the body in any one direction. Nutrients reach the body much more quickly if ingested in liquid or semi-liquid form. Additional ingredients can change the nature of *zhou*, making it an ideal vehicle to transport energies if the body needs warming, cooling, or toning in any particular area (see Chapter Seven).

Yin and *yang* foods

YIN	YANG	NEUTRAL
banana	ginger	aduki beans
crab	onion	pumpkin
kelp	garlic	Job's tears
lettuce	lamb	beancurd
celery	peach	spinach
pear	honey	sesame oil
water chestnut	shrimp	apricots
bamboo shoots	organ meats	grapes
salt	beans	plums
whole egg/egg-white	beetroot	olives
grapefruit	walnuts	aubergine
pork (mild)	egg yolk	figs
sea-grass and seaweed	chestnuts	rice

Acquiring the zhou *habit*

To make *zhou* simply simmer rice or your chosen grain in about ten times its volume of water for about forty minutes,

Traditional Chinese *zhou* is best made with a short grain white rice. The best readily available variety in the West is Arboro or risotto rice. Easy to digest, *zhou* is real comfort food, and great for late night eating. For one person you only need an egg-cup full of short grain white rice. For best results wash it well and soak it for fifteen minutes to get rid of excess starch. Then place it in a pan with ten egg cups (yes ten!) of stock or water, bring to the boil, and allow it to bubble for five minutes or so, and stir to release the starch. Simmer over a very low heat for forty minutes and the rice will absorb the liquid and reach a thin porridge consistency.

For a more substantial dish you can use other grains and thy generally don't need soaking. You can also make a richer dish by using pre-cooked grains, covering with a non-dairy milk and simmering until they reach a consistency you like.

There is always the option of oatmeal if *zhou* is a little intimidating in the first instance. An alternative to cooking grains is the traditional Swiss method of soaking muesli overnight in water. All the nutrients of the wholegrain are retained and the flavour seeps out to into the liquid to make a delicious juice, which is even tastier if enhanced with dried fruit, nuts and some desiccated coconut. There is no need to add milk; whole grains are packed with nutrients, especially when accompanied by fruits and nuts. The same cannot be said for the modern-day proprietary products that rely on the additional nutrients of milk and a large number of synthetically prepared added vitamins and minerals to allow them to make their nutrition claims. Modern breakfast cereals are simply an over-processed, over-packaged variation of the boiled grains that featured in traditional diets and which are still eaten in China

Make your own *zhou*

The best grains for *zhou*:
short grain white or brown rice • wild rice • millet • quinoa • cornmeal • Job's tears (coix seed) • buckwheat • barley

Other ingredients you might like to add:
aduki beans • mung beans • split peas or lentils • sliced Shitake mushrooms • chopped sweet potato • sweetcorn (add just before serving) • chinese dates (jujube) (see page 194) • wolfberries (sometimes sold as gouji berries) (see page 194) • dried apricots • prunes

Toppings (for savoury *zhou*):
chopped spring onion • minced coriander • chilli sauce • soy or fish sauce • sesame oil • chopped or boiled peanuts, pinenuts, walnuts • sprouted seeds (allow to soften) • fine slivers of ginger

today. During my time in China I was very sad to see the breakfast cereal manufacturers move in with a vengeance. In *The Food of China*, E. N. Anderson includes a survey of western and Chinese foods used by Chinese immigrants who had been in the US for five years.[6] It shows that two-thirds of the families surveyed had adopted the breakfast cereal and milk habit, and indicates that dry cereals were the greatest western influence on their diet after bread. The most important meal of the day is the one where there is the most time pressure, and so advertisers have spent millions convincing us of the benefits of 'special breakfast foods'. The overall eating experience is not a particularly satisfying one, despite food manufacturers' claims to the contrary, and all that salt and sugar can be habit-forming. Certainly my daily bowl of branflakes was the last vestige of my western diet, and I used to enjoy a couple of pieces of wholemeal toast with honey and a banana, all washed down with a cup of good strong English tea. In western terms these are pretty healthy options, and it is easier to form a habit than to break one. So I probably would have kept the whole idea of *zhou* on the back burner, limiting my intake to half a dozen bowls a year to humour Guo Gui Lan, had it not been made easily available to me and presented as a favourable option.

We were having breakfast at the Riverside Hotel in Hoi An, a former Vietnamese trading port famous for its mixture of cultural influences. There is excellent French bread available on the streets of Vietnam, but it had not reached our breakfast buffet – the yellow-looking buns actually tasted more like a processed cake. There was some dubious looking 'toast', but I knew that the French had never worked that one out for themselves so there wasn't much hope of their passing it on to the Vietnamese. Ignoring the children's squeals of horror and against a background of their gagging and retching noises, I decided that it was time I started eating *zhou*. Following the lead of my fellow Asian guests, I filled a small bowl with the white paste-like substance and then scattered a mixture of deep-fried garlic chips, shallots, chopped green onion, peanuts and fresh red chilli over the top, followed by a few splashes of fish sauce and sesame oil. By the third day my body had stopped wondering where the toast and honey had gone. I never looked back.

Liquid food at any time of day

When the Chinese started to mill flour in the Han dynasty (long before Marco Polo reputedly made his way along the Silk Road), they compensated for taking the moisture out of the grain by serving their noodles in liquid. In the West we eat bread with our soup; bread is baked, which makes it very dry or *yang*, and this may be why many people find it hard to digest. The Chinese make a nutritious broth using a small amount ginger and spring onion and put vegetables and noodles in it to make a one-dish meal. This traditional form of serving noodles and even dumplings is much more popular than the more modern recipes for fried noodles, and is particularly popular in the summer months.

Chinese noodles are usually made simply from wheat flour and water and come fresh, dried, hand-rolled or machine-cut and in a whole variety of shapes and thicknesses. But local stores also offer egg, spinach, buckwheat and corn noodles as well as rice noodles – which are not actually called noodles (because the Chinese name *mian tiao* means 'thin strips of flour') but *mi fen*, meaning 'tiny bits of rice'. So, if you are one of the many people in the West who suffer from wheat or gluten allergies, there are plenty of alternatives to wheat noodles.

While lacking the restorative powers of *zhou*, a bowl of noodles is nevertheless more easily accessible and quicker to make. Noodle houses were originally opened to fill the gap between formal restaurants and street food, but now offer quick inexpensive meals to people on the go. The simplest recipes use a water-based stock, flavoured with a few chunks of ginger and spring onion. Richer, more nutritious dishes can be made with a chicken stock. Toppings usually feature what is easily available: tomato and egg, minced aubergine

Noodles in soup
Tang mian

This recipe can be subject to infinite variation. Made simply with water, it is very light in flavour. You can use plain, wholemeal, buckwheat or rice noodles. For a more substantial dish add pieces of carrot or broccoli, or use a vegetable stock cube or a light chicken stock and add shredded meat and peas. For a richer dish mince the ginger and spring onion, frying them first.

1 litre/2 pints/5 cups water
100 g/3½ oz/1 cup dried noodles
a few slices of ginger
a few slices of spring onion
1 tomato, chopped into eight
2 eggs, beaten
salt to taste
1 tsp sesame oil
1 tbsp coriander leaves, roughly chopped

Add the ginger and spring onion to the water and bring to the boil. Simmer for a few minutes to allow the flavours to permeate, then add the noodles. Simmer for three minutes or until the noodles are nearly cooked. Add the tomato pieces. Trickle the eggs into the soup, pouring through chopsticks or a fork, moving around the pan to ensure that the egg pieces are well distributed. Season with salt and top with sesame oil and coriander.

Serve as soon as the egg mixture is cooked. Chinese chefs often add white pepper to give their soup a kick. You can try this, or some freshly ground black for a fusion touch.

with tiny prawns, minced green beans, dried mushrooms and bamboo shoots, or just a handful of seasonal vegetables.

The Chinese idea of liquid food may be difficult to get your head round but it is surprisingly easy to realize. Noodles are now my stock-in-trade lunch on the run, taking less time to make than to make grilled cheese on toast, and can be carried in a thermos when you are away from home.

Sadly, few moist *yin* foods are eaten regulalry in the western diet. As a sideline to my cooking school I used to help my western clients who wanted to entertain at home by putting together menus and supplying Chinese chefs. My objective was to offer something more authentic than the menus produced by the numerous embassy chefs who moonlighted at the weekends and churned out sweet and sour dishes, spring rolls and fried rice in a pineapple boat. But I found that I had my work cut out. One winter's day I was planning a meal with a Finnish woman. She reeled off a list of eight rich oily and meat-based dishes. I suggested a proliferation of vegetable alternatives but she was convinced that the male guests would not like them. Then I recommended some lighter dishes such as beef, potato and carrot stew or winter melon soup with pork balls. 'Oh no,' she told me firmly, 'those dishes aren't very Chinese.'

I knew the woman quite well. She had a flushed appearance and suffered from various skin complaints, all signs of an excess of *yang* energy. She was not overweight, because she did not eat lunch; she found it preferable to spend a large proportion of her life eating very poor-quality, mundane and tasteless food, or nothing at all, and then, splash out on a few elaborate and rich dishes, rather than, eat regular meals which used a wide range of ingredients and a mixture of cooking methods. By limiting her food intake to this type of food she was not keeping her body in balance.

If you suffer from skin complaints, headaches, nosebleeds, hot flushes or even regular outbursts of hiccups it is likely that your diet is too *yang*. Of course these may be symptoms of some deeper, underlying imbalance, but there is a fair chance that by eating more *yin* ingredients and taking in more liquid food on a regular basis you could improve your health.

Like every aspect of the Chinese diet, the fifth secret does not involve lists or calculations: just add a liquid element to every meal or at least to your daily food intake. A high proportion of liquid in your diet will help with your quest to feel satisfied after each meal yet ready to eat the next one. When you get used to eating liquid food you will find that you need to drink less, particularly at mealtimes, and you will feel more comfortable for this.

Tang soup, *zhou* and noodles are all simple to prepare, and will add another dimension to your new diet and additional opportunities to eat more and, use new and different ingredients. Enjoy them.

six

Bring *yin* and *yang* into your kitchen

'Water has the property of coldness; fire the property of heat. The interdependence of *yin* and *yang* is reflected in all things in the universe and cannot be separated.'

FROM *NEIJING SUWEN*, THE INNER CANON OF
THE YELLOW EMPEROR OR HUANGDI,
CIRCA SECOND CENTURY AD

About five years after I moved to Beijing, a branch of IKEA opened; like all ex-pats I made a beeline for it, keen to lose myself in the anonymity of the western consumer environment. At first I was amazed that so many Chinese people were in the market for designer kitchens and three-piece suites, even inexpensive ones. But as I pushed my way through the throngs though to the check-out, I noticed that most people were leaving the store with nothing more than a pack of light bulbs or a wooden photo frame. IKEA's first visitors did not come to spend money on superfluous household items, they came to look and wonder. IKEA Beijing's range of goods gradually adapted to meet the needs of the Chinese household.

Inexpensive functional items – shoe-racks, kitchen storage, fold-away tables and beds and melamine coffee tables with removable lids replaced top-end bulky ones. Six-piece saucepan sets gradually gave way to shiny woks, and dinner services to piles of ceramic rice bowls. The average Chinese kitchen is still a corridor with a single gas ring, a steel sink, with a small cupboard above.

I spent many an hour at the tiny apartment of my Chinese teacher Hong Yun, on the third ring road. We studied at the tiny bench that served her and her husband as both a desk and dining table while Sam slept obligingly on the double bed in the only other room that was deserving of the name. While Hong Yun patiently went over the finer points of Chinese grammar I marvelled at what I glimpsed through the open door to the neighbouring kitchen. There was nowhere obvious to prepare food and no store cupboard either. When I did manage to distract her attention from the lesson of the day on to this much more interesting subject she laughed and told me that her husband, who had a safe job with the government and worked regular hours, shopped every day on the way home from work and that he chopped the vegetables on the table. Where else?

A significant difference between the Chinese and western kitchen, whether traditional or modern, plays a major part in keeping the cuisine fresh, light and healthy as Mr Li Guo, the Director of the CCTV's International Channel 9, pointed out to me in my job interview.

It was a tense occasion. Sitting on an incredibly low sofa, I was relieved by my final choice of outfit, a pair of black trousers and a twinset, as coping with a rising pencil skirt, as well as answering his oblique questions, would have been far too much. 'So what do you think about Chinese food?' asked

Mr Li Guo. My immediate response, 'I love it', sounded trite and insincere. 'Do you like our programme?' came next. Never having watched it, as we didn't have a television, I told him I found it interesting, not exactly a lie as anything to do with Chinese food was of interest to me. Then came the big one: 'What do you think is the main difference between Chinese and western cooking?'

This was the question I had been waiting for and I launched into my explanation of *cai* and *fan*. I talked animatedly about the preparation involved in Chinese cooking. I waxed lyrical about how Chinese chefs really understand individual ingredients. Mr Guo listened tolerantly. 'The Chinese don't have ovens,' he said firmly. 'And can you start on Wednesday?'

A whole range of cooking methods

The multi-dish approach of a Chinese meal allows it to feature a whole range of cooking methods, as any well-balanced eating occasion always does. There is a very widely held misconception that Chinese cooking is all about stir-frying, and certainly this fast and efficient art opens up a wealth of possibilities on the culinary front – I urge you to use it more. But stir-frying is not the most commonly used method of cooking in Chinese cuisine; in fact it comes in third, after boiling and steaming. Of course a lot of rice is boiled and I have already talked about the importance of *zhou* and *tang* in the Chinese diet, but there are also all manners of stews and braised dishes, not to mention simple steamed delicacies.

Deep-fried and stir-fried, the types of dishes my Finnish friend erroneously associated with Chinese cuisine and which you will probably be familiar with are considered by Chinese people to have very *yang* characteristics and so are generally consumed in moderation. They are always balanced with *yin* dishes, which have been cooked by methods that retain moisture, such as boiling, simmering and steaming. Of course nothing is entirely *yin* or totally *yang*, and the overall characteristic of a dish will also depend on the *yin* and *yang* and the heating and cooling properties of its ingredients. As mentioned earlier, food that is *yang* ascends and disperses; it tends to have an influence on the skin, the body tissues and body surface in general. Food that is *yin* descends, to nourish and tone on the internal organs. Also, and perhaps self-evidently when you consider the different charateristics of the cooking methods, *yang* foods have a tendency to dry out the body whereas *yin* ones will moisten it.

Roasting, baking and grilling are also *yang* cooking methods, so much of the foods we eat in the West are of a *yang* nature. Bread is a prime example. I have already mentioned in Chapter Four how the Chinese steam *mantou*, some plain, some flavoured with sesame paste or ground Sichuan peppercorns; they also make cornmeal bread, either in great slabs or fashioned into little conical towers known as *wo tou*.

You are unlikely to find time to make *mantou* on a daily basis, but you don't need to. Just make sure that you are aiming for a balance in the nature of the food that you cook. This is the overwhelming theme of Chinese food culture. In China, where every meal features a soup and most staples are eaten plainly boiled or steamed, there is scope in the diet for some rich stir-fries or even deep-fried foods. If, however, your diet is based on a baked staple or, even worse, a deep-fried one, then you will need to eat a lot of steamed or boiled accompaniments. That means lots of soup with your bread, extra vegetables with your chips, or, better still, work towards the

Yin and *yang* cooking methods

Yin cooking methods:
boiling • simmering • stewing • braising • plunging (hot–pot style) • steaming

Yang cooking methods:
roasting and grilling • baking • deep-frying • stir-frying • sautéing

multi-dish approach where the rich *yang* dishes are just one part of a meal which includes plenty of *yin* options.

The need for a range of cooking methods to achieve a balance in a meal is one reason why, despite IKEA's efforts and mock-up displays, ovens have yet to catch on in China. Actually, roasted foods do feature in multi-course meals, though I was smart enough not to point this out to Mr Guo. In Hong Kong and Canton barbecued and roasted meats are great delicacies, but they are always coated and carefully seasoned because Chinese people believe that meat that is browned or burnt could potentially be damaging to health. This has also been shown in recent studies in the West.[7] And in China roasted foods are not cooked in people's homes but bought from specialist shops. Roasting or baking in an individual oven would be considered a waste of heat, and ovens would probably be used for less than half the year at most. In the stifling summer months many Chinese people favour quickly-cooked light dishes: noodles or dumplings are plunged into soup; vegetables are steamed on top of rice and then dipped in piquant sauces.

The paradox of Chinese cuisine

I spent several of my years in China living in houses where the kitchen had no oven. Friends were amazed and could not imagine how I managed. Basing a meal round a large roast, or even casserole or bake, does appear an easier option than producing lots of different dishes at the last moment. But over the years I came to find that working in a Chinese-style kitchen has its advantages, one of the greatest being that producing one dish at a time creates far less washing up.

When I presented the Chinese cooking programme for CCTV the chefs and I worked in a small windowless hotel room, furnished with nothing but an oblong white sheet clad table, a gas bottle and a burner. On the burner sat a single wok and at its side lay a chopper, a long handled spoon, a sieve and a pair of long chopsticks. The simplicity of the set-up always brought home to me the paradox of Chinese cuisine: even complex dishes can be produced with the simplest of utensils. I used to remind myself of this when I needed confidence on the culinary front, and I emphasize this to encourage you to cook new foods in new ways and not fear that that your endeavours will result in kitchen chaos.

In the TV studio, and in my cooking classes, we would pour the necessary sauces and seasonings into small bowls, complete the chopping process and arrange all ingredients for each dish together before starting to cook. Chinese cooks work in a similar way in their own homes, to ensure they are in complete control, not only of their ingredients, but of the cooking process too, so they do not end up desperately wielding the chopper or searching for sauces and seasonings at the last minute. And they never let their tiny cooking areas get disorganized or untidy. In the Chinese mind, food is always in the proper place, whether on the chopping board, in the wok or pan, or on the table. Thus cooking is never daunting, the idea of eating well is never intimidating.

The Chinese word *sheng shi* can be roughly translated as 'sensible' but also means 'appropriate'. It aptly describes the Chinese kitchen, which is never encumbered with superfluous utensils. There is no room to store unwieldy bowls and platters of differing depths and sizes, or complete sets of saucepans. Apart from a wok, most households own one flameproof glazed sand-pot and a double-handled saucepan, which will also be used as a steamer. A couple of long-handled spoons will usually hang on the wall, along with a slotted spoon, a sieve and a pair of outsized chopsticks.

The wok

Sheng shi is also a particularly apt way to describe the wok – a wide round-bottom pan, traditionally made of cast-iron whose clever design allows for maximum heat transfer with minimum use of resources. One of the reasons that Chinese meals are produced quickly and neatly is because, in the tiny Chinese domestic kitchen, the same wok is used over and over again, not just to produce the delicious stir-fries which are synonymous with Chinese food but also for blanching, boiling, steaming and simmering too.

Note that if you buy a wok with a lid and a steaming rack you can use it for almost every culinary purpose. Water comes to the boil much more quickly in a wok than in a saucepan because of its efficient design, so it is equally useful for a simple task such as poaching eggs as it is for tasty stir-fry dishes.

I have mentioned that woks are traditionally made of iron; hand-beaten cast-iron woks are still favoured by serious Chinese cooks. They do not come up clean and sparkling after washing like the new shiny stainless-steel varieties, and they will rust if not used regularly, but they are simply much better to cook with. Many modern range-style gas cookers are fitted with a wok burner; and if you are fortunate enough to have one of these then stir-frying will be a pleasure. If you don't, then think about Hong Yun's tiny burner and peservere.

Gas cookers allow you to fine-tune the heat supply to your wok, but they are not a pre-requisite for stir-frying. I have seen amazing spreads cooked on wood-fired stoves in rural China. If you are cooking on an electric stove, however, you will need to buy a flat-bottomed wok, and I have found in this situation that the non-stick variety works best.

I have already eulogized stir-fried vegetables in Chapter Two. In order to avoid your ingredients sticking to the pan or burning, always heat the wok before you add the oil; then heat the oil before tossing in the vegetables. If you are using dried chilies or Sichuan peppercorns these should be added first to flavour the oil. Minutely-chopped pieces of ginger and spring onion have a tendency to shrivel in hot oil, so I tend to add them at the same time as the vegetables; the taste still permeates the dish as the wok is very efficient at transferring flavours as well as heat.

Steaming

Mastering the art of stir-frying will greatly enhance your culinary repertoire, but do also keep coming back to the issue of balance and experiment with other new ways of cooking. Steaming is a great way to prepare moist and nutritious dishes. Fish is particularly suited to steaming, as are root vegetables including sweet potatoes, and the nutritious yam known as *shan yao* ('mountain medicine'). In China, steamed aubergines are mashed with garlic and sesame to make a pungent dip reminiscent of the Middle Eastern *babaganoush*; steamed pumpkin is drizzled with garlickly oil; tofu pieces are stuffed with slivers of bamboo shoots and Shitake mushroom, then steamed until the flavours merge. Most modern Chinese kitchens now boast a rice cooker and, in another example of how Chinese cooking is *sheng shi*, many Chinese cooks place vegetables, morsels of meat or Chinese sausage on top of the rice, to steam while it cooks and flavour the rice at the same time. This can be done either on a special steaming basket or by opening the cooker part way through cooking and placing the ingredient directly on the rice.

Plunging

Another very simple but delicious way of eating that is popular throughout China, though with regional variations, is the hot-pot, whereby slivers of meat or fish, slices of beancurd and a plethrora of vegetables are plunged into boiling stock or water, removed with chopsticks and then dipped into one of several accompaniments. A particularly sociable way of eating, it is also easy to prepare at home. The Beijing favourite is a combination of wafer-thin lamb, cabbage, cellophane noodles and beancurd, with a spicy sesame paste dip. But you can prepare any combination of ingredients that you enjoy.

Stewing and braising

In rural areas, stews and braised dishes simmer on wood or coal-fired stoves, the same ones that are used, in winter to heat the water for the household. Specially designed pans fit onto the burners so that no heat escapes and food can be cooked using a minimum amount of fuel, creating dishes that are low in oil and high in nutrients. City dwellers in their modern apartments have become accustomed to their single gas ring, but the traditional importance of the stove in Chinese culture is illustrated by the fact that the kitchen god is said to reside within it.

Very few of the rich repertoire of Chinese stews have ever made it to the West. When meat is stewed in China it is almost always left on the bone for maximum flavour and nutrition, and western diners often find this off-putting. Stews are usually made in sand-pots, traditional earthenware bowls, glazed on the outside but with a creamy, unglazed texture on the inside. Porous and heat-retardant, they add a delicate flavour of past meals to every stew. And each new dish is packed full of esoteric ingredients, from cellophane noodles to mushrooms and fungus and from dried beancurd to lotus root and seeds. They also feature pungent spices including variations on the famous 'five-spice',[8] which, contrary to what is often taught in the West is a seasoning used for marinades and stews, not for stir-frying. Ingredients such as star anise, cinnamon, hawthorn, orange-peel, red dates and wolfberries (known in

Beef and potato stew
Tu dou dun niu rou

This simple stew is packed full of health-giving ingredients yet incredibly simple to make. If you cannot find all the spices listed just use the ones that you have. In the north of China people sometimes add dried chilies or Sichuan peppercorns too.

500 g/1 lb/3 cups diced organic beef skirt
(the more sinew the better)
1 spring onion, cut into four or five lengths
2 cm/1in piece ginger, crushed
6 slices dried red hawthorn
6 slices dried orange peel
3 pieces of star anise
1 stick cinnamon
1 bay leaf
splash of Chinese cooking wine
2 tbsp soy sauce
½ tsp salt (or to taste)
1 potato, peeled and cubed
1 carrot, peeled and cubed

Put the beef into a saucepan or casserole pot. Cover with cold water and add a splash of cooking wine. Bring the water to the boil and skim off any scum that collects on the surface. If you cannot get rid of all the scum you can change the water.

Add the spices (but not the salt and the soy sauce) and turn the heat down to a simmer for half an hour. Then add the soy sauce and simmer for another hour. Finally add the salt, potato and carrot, and simmer for a further half hour until the vegetables are cooked.

China as *gou qi zi* and sold in the West as *goji* or *gouji* berries) are all commonly used to make the meat in Chinese stews immensely flavoursome and either to help make it tender and easy to digest, or greatly enhance the nutrient value of the mix.

The British equivalent of a stove is of course an Aga but if you do not have a farmhouse kitchen, a slow or pressure cooker will help you prepare simmered dishes in a western context. The good old fashion stew has slipped from favour in recent years, as richer, more visually appealing dishes have reached our tables. But you can add interest to your pot with Asian spices and give stew another lease of life, especially if you present it as just one element of an interesting meal. The preparation is minimal: just chop up your ingredients, put them in the pot, cover with liquid and bring to the boil.

Braising involves frying or sautéing before simmering, so is more *yang* than stewing. This may be why it is favoured for vegetable dishes. Cabbage, bamboo shoots, Shitake mushrooms, aubergine and potato all braise very successfully Chinese style. The Chinese way tends to be to braise one main vegetable at a time, an approach that has many advantages. I love to braise red and yellow peppers with cumin and paprika, or beetroot with chilli and coconut. If you want to braise a mixture of vegetables, perhaps with Indian seasonings, then you may have to check cooking times to ensure that some do not become mushy before the others are cooked through.

Yin *and* yang *—a truly balanced diet*

The multi-dish, *cai* and *fan* approach of Chinese cooking is ultimately flexible and can make for quick and easy eating.

The various cooking methods can all be carried out in a basic kitchen with a handful of utensils. A stew or steamed dish can be in the process of cooking, usually in the dish in which it will be served, while the chef concentrates on the other dishes, one at a time. There is never any pressure to bring everything together at the last moment as dishes can be put on the table in any order. If you are often overwhelmed by multiple gadgets, pots and serving vessels, or find yourself constantly refering to recipe books while keeping one eye on the timer and frantically stirring a sauce, consider taking a more Chinese approach in your kitchen.

seven

Balance the flavours

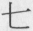

'I consider that the mouth and the stomach do more harm than good. It was mistake for nature to endow us with them.'

LI YU (1611–1680)

The seventeenth-century poet Li Yu warned his public about the risk of listening only to the preferences of the mouth and stomach, and not the rest of the body. He suggests that 'since we are stuck with our mouth and stomach we will have them serve our purposes instead of serving them.'

I spent many an hour huddled in an overcoat sipping green tea, in a dingy lecture room at the Beijing Hospital of Traditional Chinese Medicine, before I fully understood the meaning of Li Yu's quote. My interest was first piqued at the close of one particular cooking class, which had been attended by a number of large ladies who all professed to eat like mice and had just signed up for a rigorous programme with a personal trainer. After they had left Xiao Ding commented in a matter-of-fact manner that the reason so many westerners have weight problems is because they eat too many sweet foods. I was surprised, as I had never previously heard her make the connection between overconsumption of any type of food and weight gain. Why, I wondered, should sweet foods be an issue when calories are not?

The seventh secret of the Chinese diet is that it features five flavours that each need to be incorporated into every meal, whenever possible. According to Chinese dietary therapy, which is a branch of Traditional Chinese Medicine, each of the five flavours of foods has a different action, and the action of 'sweet' foods is related to the mouth and stomach, which is why we should not eat too many of them. Of course, we all know that if we put too much in our mouths, it ends up round our stomach, especially if we indulge our preferences, started in childhood, for sweets and treats. But Chinese dietary therapy defines 'sweet' very differently from the way we do in the West.

The meaning of 'sweet'

There are many 'sweet' foods found in nature: honey is obviously sweet, but so are carrots, sweetcorn, figs and watermelon. In theory it would be difficult to overload on these foods. The modern diet tricks nature with sugar-loaded sweets, puddings, cakes and biscuits, and we are all aware of the dangers of eating too many of these foods. But many people following restrictive slimming diets that cut out these obvious 'baddies' still find themselves unable to shift their excess weight. This is, according to Chinese dietary therapy, because their diet is still not balanced in terms of the five flavours. Instead, it is largely made up of rather bland foods, which in the absence of any more obvious flavour, and because of the way they are seen to affect the body, are also regarded as 'sweet'.

The first step to appreciating the teachings of Traditional Chinese Medicine is to understand that it does not consider the body as an anatomical entity but as a series of energy centres. According to the Taoist concept, which has helped man work in harmony with nature for thousands of years, the world is made up of Five Elements: wood, fire, earth, metal and water. These have a complex interdependence and are everywhere and in everything, including the human body, where they manifest themselves in the energy centres or organs. There are five pairings of organs: the spleen/stomach, the liver/gall-bladder, the heart/small intestine, the lungs/large intestine and the kidney/bladder. These should be distinguished from their counterparts in western biological science because, while parallels can be drawn, they work in a much more holistic way and are endowed with many attributes and functions that western science does not recognize. One of these is that they are linked to five orifices: the liver is linked to the eye, the heart to the tongue, the lung to the nose, the kidney to the ear. Not surprisingly, the stomach/spleen is linked to the mouth – and here lies the basis for Li Yu's opinion.

According to Chinese dietary therapy, and the Five Elements scheme of things, there are five flavours of foods: sweet, sour, salty, pungent and bitter and each one 'enters' one of the five pairs of organs. Thus the sweet flavour enters the spleen/stomach. The sour flavour finds its way into the liver/gall-bladder, the bitter enters the heart/small intestine, the pungent enters the lung/large intestine and the salty flavour enters the kidney/bladder. While the right amount of a flavour tones and benefits an organ, too much will damage it and hinder it from performing its functions.

ELEMENT	wood	fire	earth	metal	water
ORGAN	liver/ gall- bladder	heart/ small intestine	spleen/ stomach	lungs/ large intestine	kidneys/ bladder
ORIFICE	eyes	tongue	mouth	nose	ear

2. The Five Elements, or Phases, the Five Pairs of Organs and the Five Orifices.

In most cases the mouth seeks out sweet-tasting foods from among the options; breast milk is sweet, and that's where it all starts; the mouth instinctively seeks out the bland macro-nutrient foodstuffs that fill the stomach and form the basis of a balanced diet. In the natural world, though, we have a resource that encompasses all the flavours, from sour fruits to bitter roots and from spicy scallions to salty seaweeds, and they all have an important role to play in toning the organs and keeping the body healthy. Our modern diet seems to offer tremendous choice but it is actually becoming increasingly limited as we tend to eat what is easily available or convenient to prepare, and to allow our mouths to follow their preference.

If we indulge in overly sweet flavours at the expense of the others, which are needed to tone the organs and keep them in balance, our digestive systems and waistbands get out of kilter, or, literally, stretched to their limits. And if one organ is out of balance, this upsets the equilibrium in our whole body. Obesity, according to Chinese medicine is just one

SOUR	LIVER/GALL-BLADDER
BITTER	HEART/SMALL INTESTINE
SWEET	SPLEEN/STOMACH
PUNGENT	LUNGS/LARGE INTESTINE
SALTY	KIDNEY/BLADDER

3. The Five Flavours enter the Five Pairs of Organs.

manifestation of an imbalance that prevents the body from thriving. Totally interdependent, the organs are linked by meridians or lines of energy that transport the *Qi*, or life-force. Good health depends on the smooth flow of *Qi* round the body, and this in turn depends on the proper functioning of the organs. In a healthy body, the organs work in harmony; if one or more of them is not working properly then ill-health, or sometimes just that feeling of 'being out of sorts' which so many people in the West accept as a fact of life, will ensue.

So the seventh secret of the Chinese diet is that 'sweet' (or bland) foods need to be complemented by foods with other flavours in order to keep the body fit and in shape. Most food flavours are easy to detect: soy sauce is salty, as is seaweed; lemons are sour; ginger, garlic spring onion, chilli and pepper are all pungent; while vinegar is sour and bitter. The need to balance the flavours in the diet is yet another reason to eat a greater number of vegetables, and fruits too, since, unlike meats and carbohydrate foods, which have a tendency to be bland, they provide a range of flavours, often combining more than one.

Asparagus, for instance, is slightly pungent and bitter, celery and lettuce are bitter and sweet, tomato, grapefruit and kiwi are sweet and sour.

I list below the flavours of some common foods. You should be able to grasp some general principles from the table (see page 98), but as a rough guide remember the following:

- Macronutrient and other bland tasting foods are generally sweet.
- Herbs and spices are generally pungent.
- Water-based foods are often salty.
- Many fruits are sour (and usually sweet too).
- Only a limited number of foods eaten regularly in the West are bitter (which is probably why most medicines are – to restore the balance).
- Balance can also be achieved during cooking, as you will see in the next chapter.

'Wait a minute!' you are thinking, 'If you tell me that cakes and biscuits, ice-creams and chocolate bars are making me fat I might accept it, but your list of "sweet" foods includes lots of "healthy" ones: peas, mushrooms, cashew nuts – even rice. Surely I am not supposed to cut those out of my diet?' But you might recall that up to this point I have not talked about cutting anything out of your diet. On the contrary, I have recommended that you enjoy your food and eat more, but I have also encouraged you to eat and learn to cook a much wider variety of foods. Under no circumstances should you stop eating peas, or mushrooms and certainly not cashew nuts or rice: all these foods can benefit health.

The nature of Chinese cooking is such that sweet or bland flavours are seldom served alone but always complemented by

SOUR	BITTER	SWEET	PUNGENT	SALTY
apple*	asparagus	banana	chives	barley*
apricot*	celery*	beancurd	chilies	clam
grapes*	bitter gourd	beef, chicken	coriander	crab
grapefruit*	dried orange-peel	butter	fennel	duck
hawthorn fruit*	hops	cabbage	ginger	ham
lemon (very)	kohlrabi (pungent and sweet)	carrot	garlic	kelp
olives*	lettuce*	eggs	spring onion	mussels
peach*	pork and sheep liver*	figs	kohlrabi	oysters
pineapple*	tea*	milk	leeks	pork*
plum*	cocoa	mushrooms	marjoram	seaweed
raspberry*		potato	mint	seagrass
small red bean (aduki)*		rice	pumpkin*	
tangerines*		shrimp	red and green peppers*	
tomato*		sweet potato	rosemary	
		watermelon	sweet basil	
The foods marked * also have a sweet flavour				

4. The Five Flavours of common foods.

spices and seasoning that represent the other flavours. The Chinese palate expects a balance, so, until recently, had little taste for the overly-sweet flavours of modern confectionary or ice-cream. Chinese cooking often features small amounts of sugar in recipes to bring out the intrinsic sweet flavour of an ingredient such as tomato, sweetcorn or even beef.

If you have been striving to achieve that feeling of satisfaction that I keep mentioning, but have not yet achieved it, your body may be telling you that it has not received everything it needs from your choice of foods. While it is quite acceptable for 'sweet' macronutrient foods to comprise the bulk of a diet, they need to be complemented by sour, pungent, bitter and salty foods, too. A diet that is balanced according to the flavours cannot fail to be one which is full of variety and packed with nutrients.

This may be why, after finishing Chinese-style meals, most diners do not have the same desire for a sweet course as we do in the West; the stomach has been satisfied, and, because of the mix of flavours in the meal, the other organs have been toned as well. This feeling of satisfaction and well-being is very different from the sensation of being full, or even 'stuffed', that often accompanies a large western meal, where the stomach may be full but the body is not in balance. On the few occasions that Chinese meals do feature a dessert-style dish it is not served at the end but is just another element in a balanced meal. A delicacy particularly enjoyed during the lantern festival which takes place at the end of the Chinese New Year week is *tang yuan*, small balls made of glutinous rice flour and stuffed with all manner of delicacies, from sesame seeds to red bean paste to chocolate; another is *basi pingguo*, a sort of hot toffee-apple. My children love this, and never complain when it arrives on the table midway through a meal.

More about Qi

To understand the importance of balancing the flavours we have to consider the flow of *Qi*, or life-force. This comes in many different forms, but is essentially made up of the air we breathe, the food we eat, and an element inherited from our parents. It is not always easy to choose the air we breathe, though we can ensure that we exercise regularly. Nor can we alter our genetic make-up, though we can make the most of our strengths. In modern society, however, we have a large degree of control over our diet.

A brief description of how the organs work in Traditional Chinese Medicine may help you to understand how important it is to eat a balance of flavours, and why, in the Chinese mind, two foods would never be judged equal just because they have the same calorie content. The spleen and stomach work together to extract the *Qi* from the food and to sort out pure *Qi*, which can be used, from the impure, which has to be excreted. The lungs take in *Qi* from the air, again separating pure from impure. The *Qi* from the lungs then combines with the *Qi* from the spleen/stomach and is sent to the heart, which is responsible for changing it into blood and then pumping it through the body. In Traditional Chinese Medicine blood has a wider meaning than just the red stuff circulating through our veins because, among other things, it carries *Qi* around the body. If your blood is weak or not flowing freely, which is quite likely if you have poor eating habits, it will be difficult for you to control your weight and you will be constantly exhausted.

The function of the kidneys in Traditional Chinese Medicine is very different from western medicine as they are regarded as the source of a different type of *Qi*, which is believed to be inherited and equated with genetic make-up. They are also the source of *jing*. A difficult concept to grasp, usually translated as 'essence', *jing* is the fundamental substance and source of living organisms and also produces bone-marrow, which is associated with the brain. *Jing* underpins *Qi*, especially the *Qi* of the kidneys. The *Qi* from the kidneys helps the heart change *Qi* into blood, which in turn carries *jing* around the body as well as *Qi*. The liver then regulates the amount of blood in circulation, thus ensuring the smooth flow of *Qi* round the body.

Recognizing the relationship between the Five Flavours and the Five Organs is the key to understanding why the Chinese diet is so satisfying. People who are overweight, or indeed underweight, often lack energy because their overloaded stomachs cannot do their job of extracting *Qi* from food, resulting in their suffering a host of niggling ailments, bloating, indigestion, constipation, lethargy and, of course, obesity.

Why Chinese people hug trees

In the early morning Chinese parks are full of people taking in the morning air. Often you will see an old woman with her leg at right angles against a tree or a man doing pull-ups. Some use one of the exercise areas that now feature in every park, but they often prefer the connection with nature – wood, in particular, represents the liver, which needs to be kept toned so that it can ensure the steady flow of blood, *Qi* and *jing*. It was only when I began to appreciate the Taoist view of the world as a living organism, where man is an integral part of a greater whole, that I began to see how every aspect of Chinese life is connected with nature and is manifest in the Five Elements of wood, fire, earth, metal and water.

The relationship between the Five Organs is best understood against the background of the Five Elements which nourish each other and consume each other all the time in what is sometimes called the 'cycle of promotion and consumption'. So the growth of *wood* is fed by *water*, but *wood* has to consume *water* to grow; *fire* is fed by *wood*, but *wood* is destroyed by *fire's* flames; *earth* is nourished by the ashes from *fire*, but *fire* can be extinguished by *earth*; *metal* comes from the *earth* but when *metal* is extracted it robs the *earth* of its resources; and *water* is divined by *metal*, but *metal* can be diluted by *water*.

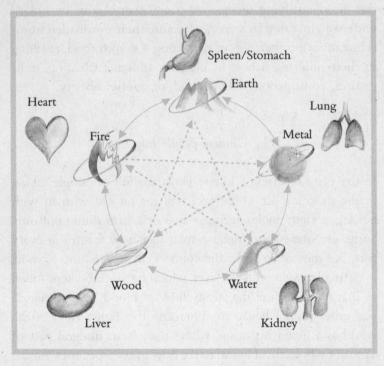

5. The Cycle of Promotion, Consumption (solid lines) and Control (broken lines).

As well as this cycle of promotion and consumption, the Five Elements also have a control cycle whereby an element can 'enter' another to tone it. Water, in its role as controller, can dampen fire, wood can smother the earth, fire can melt metal, earth can absorb water, and metal can enter and cut the wood. All elements need to be toned to keep the balance of the cycle. But the controller must not be too strong or it will damage the element it enters.

The Five Elements correspond to, and are seen as being within, the Five Organs. Thus *wood* has a special relationship with the liver, *fire* with the heart, *earth* with the spleen/stomach, *metal* with the lung and *water* with the kidneys. We may use the Five Elements cycle to get a better understanding of what happens when we eat the wrong foods. If an excess of *sweet* flavour enters the spleen/stomach (*earth*) it may at first make it too strong but ultimately it will damage it. An over-nourished *earth* element may smother *fire*, a weak one may let it get out of control. And when *earth* is weak it cannot promote *metal* nor regulate *water*. Overloading the spleen/stomach will affect the heart, the lungs and kidneys. Practically all the ailments that beset the West, from heart disease to asthma and water retention can all be traced back to maltreatment of the spleen/stomach in the first instance. Just as the elements and the organs create and control each other in the Five Elements cycle, so do the flavours. The right amount of a flavour will keep an organ toned so that it is neither too strong nor too weak. An excess or a shortage will eventually damage it and let it take the rest of the body down with it.

This relationship explains a little more about our dietary preferences and what we need to beware of. The young growth

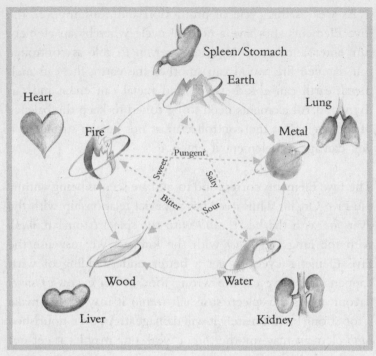

6. The Five Flavours in the Five Elements Cycle.

of *wood* is *sweet*, *salt* comes from the *earth*; *fire* is *pungent*; *metal*, like the *sour* flavour, is astringent; *water* has no flavour but can leave a *bitter* taste.

The human lifecycle can also be seen in terms of the Five Elements. When we are young we are in the *wood* stage, growing fast. The *fire* stage represents the late teenage years and young adulthood. *Earth* corresponds to the nurturing period, when we settle down. By the *metal* stage we have begun to contract our lives. Finally, *water* represents the stillness of old age and eventual death. When we are young our *wood* element is in ascendancy and we have a natural affinity for *sweet* flavours, but it is the *sour* flavour from *metal* that actually enters and tones the liver. Children, therefore, should not overindulge in sweet things but be tempted with sour fruits instead. In our teenage years the *fire* element and the heart are dominant. Teenagers often develop a taste for hot foods, both spicy and warming in terms of the energies mentioned earlier, but actually they need to go easy on the curry and chocolate and favour the bitter flavours of greens and vinegary dressings, and plenty of water. These will tone their *fire* element and keep it under control; otherwise they will suffer from acne, restlessness and other heat–related conditions.

The body can often accommodate bad eating habits during the wood and fire stages, but it is in the earth phase, at the prime of our life that we are at greatest risk of putting on weight because the spleen/stomach is in ascendancy and *earth* does not grow or move as in the previous phases. Unlike sour and bitter, which are in short supply in many diets, *sweet* flavour needs to be restricted while its organ is in ascendancy.

As we get older and enter the metal stage of our lives we should become more discerning and eat less but better, with plenty of the pungent flavours that enter the lungs: this is the time when we really need foods with active constituents such as garlic, ginger, chilies and other herbs and spices. The *water* element, linked to the kidneys, is in ascendancy as we enter old age. The *salty* flavour enters the kidneys from the *earth* element; but the salty foods that benefit the body are natural ones – kelp, seaweed, and many types of seafood. If we have overindulged in too much unnaturally salty food because we have eaten a diet high in processed foods during our youth, we could suffer as we get older. Remember that in Traditional Chinese Medicine, the kidneys are the source of the *Qi*, our life-force, and *jing*, our essence, which is believed to be the source of all life. In our last years we may need to seek out the bitter flavours of foods with medicinal properties if we want to survive into old age.

The role of rice

How does all this translate into practical terms? As Li Yu remarked all those years ago, the worst thing we can do is pander to the mouth and stomach. A French student once approached me in my cooking school. Her husband, she explained, had struggled with his weight for years. His job was stressful and sedentary, and not only was he overweight but his digestion was bad, and that was affecting his morale. Western dietary regimes only added to his stress since they put so much emphasis on exercise routines that he didn't feel up to. She was constantly measuring and calorie-counting and preparing special dishes: did I have any suggestions?

When I looked at her husband's diet sheets I felt sorry for both of them. Their whole regimen consisted of steamed fish, grilled chicken breast, carefully measured scrapings of butter on accurately-weighed pieces of bread. There were a few token vegetables, though without any suggestions as to how to make them interesting, and a thimbleful of milk to share between the unlimited rations of tea and coffee.

I suggested that she should base their meals on vegetables, provide unlimited rice, use a range of cooking methods and, most importantly, balance the flavours in every meal. And because we were in China where culinary skills are practically universal, I found a friend of Xiao Ding's, Xiao Li, who was willing to help her cook in this new style. At first everything went as well as could be expected. My friend's husband, Antoine, had a few problems adjusting to the more fibrous nature of his new diet, but he generally felt better in himself and was thrilled to be freed from the burden of calorie-counting. My friend was ecstatic, though she was slightly overwhelmed by the quantity of food that her helper produced. After a few weeks, however, her husband's progress ground to a halt. 'He misses his French diet too much,' she explained. I sympathized. 'Especially the desserts,' she continued. This was surprising, since I had envisaged that, with a diet offering a full spectrum of flavours, Antoine would lose interest in very sweet foods. When I probed I discovered that, although he was eating the Chinese dishes in the evenings and usually taking leftovers with him for lunch, he was not eating the rice. Warning bells clanged in my head. While I saw that a variety of vegetables and a balance of flavours to be the key to nourishing the whole body through the Chinese diet, without a staple I couldn't see how it would be sustaining. From observing how Chinese people ate I knew that *fan* was the food that filled the stomach and stopped it craving sweet flavours. The seventh secret of the Chinese diet is supported by the third secret: *fan* is the foundation on which the Five-Flavour balance rests. This is why the Five Element chart is sometimes drawn with earth at its centre. Unless Antoine could escape his western prejudices and fill up on a staple food, I knew he would not benefit in the long term from his change to a more Chinese-style diet.

In our modern society, where foods are often judged in terms of their calorific content, little account is taken of the flavours of foods and how they work together within the body. Yet our western tastebuds are not beyond rescue – curry, after all, is the UK's favourite dish. The sweet, sour and spicy flavours of *gong bao ji ding*, a chicken and peanut dish, never failed to impress my cooking school students. The same flavours are found in the Sichuan *yu xiang qie zi* aubergine recipe. Now, *yu xiang* translates as 'fish fragrant', which sounds a bit off-putting, but the story goes that the recipe, which is sweet, sour and spicy with a slight fermented flavour from *dou ban jiang* (chilli bean paste), was developed in landlocked Sichuan to compensate for the absence of fish on the menu. There are *yu xiang* dishes featuring pork and eggs, but the aubergine with strips of pork and cloud-ear mushrooms takes some beating. If you serve a *gong bao ji ding* and a *yu xiang qie zi* plus a stir-fried green vegetable topped with plenty of freshly chopped garlic and a bowl of rice to anyone brought up on a western diet, they'll think they have been invited to a feast.

Simple touches can transform more conventional western dishes. The Mexicans add grated bitter chocolate to their stews; pork is served with pungent mustard sauce; mint is added to pea soup, fresh lemon juice is squeezed on to fish. You do not need to deny yourself any favourites in order to improve your diet according to the principles of balancing flavours. Try instead to start by adding a depth of flavour to your traditional meals. Serve sweet and sour red cabbage with raisins, apple and Balsamic vinegar with your roast; grate the cheese for your sandwiches and mix it with minced celery. Once you start to add variety to your diet, and let Chinese cuisine influence your cooking, traditional western food may seem bland and indigestible. During my time in China I saw my own diet change from one consisting primarily of bland or sweet food to one with the full range of flavours. So, if you are struggling with a chocolate craving or a passion for Häagen-Dazs, don't fight it. Adopt the Chinese style of eating and it will eventually go away of its own accord as the new range of flavours in your diet helps the body discover its own natural balance.

Spicy chicken with peanuts
Gong bao ji ding

恭爆鸡丁

This Sichuan dish is an all time classic and is often known overseas by its Cantonese name, Kung Pao chicken. Sadly, the recipe has been abused as much as used, and there are some extraordinary variations about. The true Sichuan version has crisp (*cui*) peanuts contrasting with tiny cubes of succulent chicken. It uses dried chilies, Sichuan peppercorns and pieces of hearty garlic, ginger and spring onion. These robust flavours are backed up by a delicate sauce with a touch of sweet and sour.

For the chicken
300 g/10 oz/2 cups organic chicken breast meat
75 g/3 oz/¾ cup roasted peanuts
2 tsp beaten egg or egg white
3 tsp cornflour
pinch of salt
1 tsp cooking wine

Supporting vegetables
1 tbsp spring onion, chopped vertically then cut into
1 cm/½ in pieces
3–4 cloves garlic, sliced
4–6 fine slices ginger, each cut into quarters
3–6 dried red chilies, roughly chopped
1 tsp Sichuan peppercorns

For the sauce mix
2 tsp soy sauce
2 tsp sugar
3 tsp red rice vinegar
1 tsp cooking wine

1–2 tbsp of a 1–2 cornflour and water mix
1–2 tbsp additional water
salt to taste
1½ tbsp oil

Cube the chicken breast, aiming for pieces which are not much bigger than the nuts. Sprinkle them with salt and cooking wine and mix well with the egg or egg white and cornflour, making sure that the pieces are coated but not sloppy.

Mix together the sauce ingredients.

To cook, heat the wok to a high heat, add the oil, swirl around, and fry the chilies and Sichuan peppercorns for a few minutes until fragrant. Add the chicken, garlic, ginger and spring onion. Stir-fry these to allow the flavour out, then add the peanuts.

Add the liquid ingredients (stirring first to dissolve the cornflour) and allow it to come to the boil stirring gently. Let the sauce simmer for a few minutes, to thicken, and then add additional liquid until the sauce reaches the desired consistency. Add extra salt to taste, mix well, remove from the heat and serve.

eight
Master your ingredients

八

'Every ingredient has its own special qualities just as different persons are differently endowed.'

YUAN MEI (1716–98)

A visiting chef once cooked pig's feet for my children's tea. I had asked him to teach me authentic Chinese dishes, so when the pink trotters emerged from his backpack there was no way I could say, 'I don't think so.' I didn't pay much attention as he simmered the offending articles in a rich *hong shao* (red braised) sauce with its sugar, soy sauce and plenty of ginger, thinking that his other two dishes of chicken wings in red wine and pan fried tofu stuffed with prawns would be much more useful to me.

When the children arrived home the dish was on the table where I usually left a snack for them. Expecting cries of horror, I said nothing and to my amazement Christian picked one up and started to chew. When he asked me later if Mr Wang would be cooking for us every night, I asked whether he'd like that. He replied that the food had been tasty but 'just a bit unusual'.

We are conditioned by our environment: I'm sure the average frankfurter contains far more unmentionable bits of pig than the trotter, but it is well disguised by processing with a good dollop of emulsifiers which make fat look like meat. The biggest difference between China and the West is not that the Chinese eat a simple diet based on rice and vegetables and we don't, or even that the Chinese eat unmentionable things and we don't; it's that the Chinese approach rice, vegetables and unmentionable things – even pig's feet – with confidence because they have the skills to make the most weird and wonderful ingredients into a dish full of balance and harmony.

The eighth secret, then, is to approach your ingredients and your cooking with creativity and confidence. If you can do so you will be able to revitalize your relationship with food. To teach you all the many technicalities of Chinese cookery is outside the scope of this book, and I have already explained that you do not need to eat a totally Chinese diet to benefit from the secrets of the Chinese food culture. But a basic understanding of the principles of Chinese cuisine will help you to choose your ingredients, prepare them in your kitchen and cook them into meals that make your whole body feel good because they appeal to all the senses.

To cook but also to select

The Chinese word for cuisine is *pengtiao*, meaning 'to cook' but also 'to select'. The first step in the selection process is a trip to the market. A Chinese chef would never take a shopping list, or start with a recipe. Instead, aware of what vegetables are in season at that time of year, he chooses the best produce on offer that day. Then he considers the qualities of the foods he has bought and decides how he will cut, season, cook and combine them.

Working from recipes is tedious and time-consuming. If you take the Chinese approach and start by buying what is fresh and in season then finding a way to make it taste good, either on its own or in simple combinations, you will gradually acquire confidence. Handling foods in this way is a very different experience from starting from a recipe and working backwards. Take courgettes, for example, something I have always used frequently in ratatouille or stuffed or in bakes, without really feeling I knew how to cook them or appreciate their many qualities. Then one day I overheard an exchange in the local market.

'What do you call those?'

'*Xi hulu*' ('western gourd': they were still relatively new to China).

'So how do you cook them?'

'You can put them in soups or stews, but they don't have much taste so are best stir-fried; halve them, cut them into slices and fry with ginger and dried chilli – they are good to eat.'

The customer bought a bagful, as did several others who had been listening in to this exchange. I followed suit and cooked them as instructed; needless to say they were good to eat. You may not get such creative advice at your local supermarket checkout (I actually find that the store assistants usually ask me about the exotic vegetables that I buy) but there are other sources in the West. I subscribe to a local 'box' scheme, which not only delivers seasonal vegetables but also provides simple but tasty recipe suggestions, recovered, I imagine, from country kitchens.

In a food culture where nothing is wasted, Chinese cooks have had to be resourceful and inventive. But they have been fortunate to live in a society where expertise is still handed down from generation to generation, as well as having thousands years of recorded history to help them. *Shi jing*, or food manuals, have been produced in China since ancient times. By the sixth century the Chinese government was sponsoring the distribution of these early cookbooks to help people make the best of local produce. Book printing, which was invented in China about 800 years earlier than it appeared in the West, made important information about food and diet easily accessible. The expertise of generations was accumulated and, as it is usual for extended family members to work together in the kitchen, this continues to be passed on.

Chinese chefs and cooks recognize that each ingredient has an intrinsic quality: the chef's task is to find a way to bring this out. The first thing he looks for is *xiang* (fragrance), a characteristic associated with freshness. The food of the southern Chinese, with its abundance of greenery, is particularly known for being *xiang*; but any ingredient that needs only gentle cooking and light seasoning is worthy of the name.

The five characteristics of a Chinese meal

- *Xiang* – Fragrance
- *Wei'r* – Taste
- *Xing* – Shape
- *Se* – Colour
- *Kou gan* – Texture (literally 'mouth feel')

As we have already seen, the Chinese place great importance on eating a diet which represents the five flavours of
food. The chef has to ensure that these are not indiscrimi-
nately combined and that each dish as has a delicious overall
taste, or *wei'r*. So when he is shopping he will look for ingredients that go well together. Chinese people use the phrase
hao chi ('good eat') all the time, and are not averse to describing
something as *bu hao chi* ('not good eat') if applicable. The
Chinese cook strives, therefore, to make every dish tasty, either
by bringing out the natural flavour of an ingredient or by
appropriate seasoning.

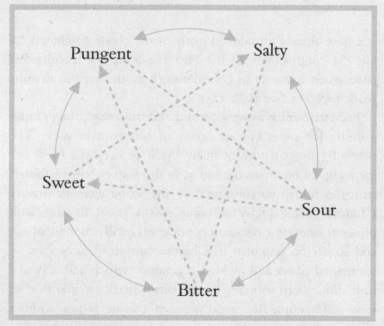

7. The Five Flavours cycle.
Solid lines show the promotion and consumption cycle, broken lines
show the control cycle.

味

> Sour tones sweet, and is toned by pungent
>
> Bitter tones pungent, and is toned by salty
>
> Sweet tones salty, and is toned by sour
>
> Pungent tones sour, and is toned by bitter
>
> Salty tones bitter, and is toned by sweet

8. How the Five Flavours affect each other.

I have already introduced many of the classic combinations, but the control cycle of the Five Elements is a useful reference when it comes to considering how the various flavours work together (see page 115).

Each flavour has a promoter and a consumer; so, bitter creates a desire for sweet but an excess of bitter masks sweet. The overlying sweet nature of many snack or breakfast foods call for a cup of bitter strong coffee, as the water element (bitter) struggles not to be consumed by the wood element (sweet). Chinese people prefer to complement sweet flavours with pungent ones. If a dish is too pungent, small amounts of salt and sugar can tranform it. Chinese cuisine features a lot of fermented pastes and pickled vegetables, which add salty and sour dimensions to many dishes. Bitter herbs are also used in stews and soups. But good western cuisine is not without effective flavour combinations: take skate with black butter (sour and bitter) and capers (salty) or a honey and mustard dressing: sweet, pungent, salty, bitter and sour.

Controlling the flavours

So, according to the control cycle, each flavour is best enhanced or tempered by two others. These do not have to be exclusive, of course – in the Five Element scheme of things all the flavours have a role to play in maintaining balance and harmony. Also remember that balance applies not only to the individual dish but to the whole meal (see page 116).

The sour flavour naturally enters sweet and is beautifully offset by the pungent flavour that enters sour. Hence the overwhelming popularity of the hot, sweet-and-sour *gong bao ji ding* in my cooking school. And the same flavours are found in *dhansak* or *patia* Indian curries. Some of the combinations in the Five-Element control cycle are not easily accessible to the western chef. If you are fortunate enough to live near to an area with specialist shops you may be able to buy *ku gua*, the Chinese bitter melon that looks like a light green cucumber, and fermented black bean paste. In China the sliced bitter melon is stir-fried with the black bean paste and sliced green chilli, resulting in an amazing bitter, salty and pungent dish. Much simpler, but equally delicious, is grated kohlrabi with chilli oil and salt. Good traditional western food can feature the control cycle too: take liver and onions (slightly bitter, pungent and salty) and the many sweet and sour chutneys that English country cooking was once famous for.

It is not difficult to incorporate the flavours in home-cooked dishes. Look for traditional recipes that use sour fruits such as redcurrants, rhubarb and of course lemons; and use the rind, too, for a bitter touch; or experiment with Indian and other flavoursome Asian ingredients using new and different spices.

You will find that if you understand the relationship between the flavours you can remedy mistakes in cooking by adding

Strange flavoured sauce
Guai wei'r jiang

怪味儿酱

This sauce is usually used to top poached shredded chicken mixed with spring onions, but it may also be used as a dip or sauce for cold noodles or as a dressing for lettuce (on the few occasions that Chinese people eat raw foods they always dress them with a spicy sauce).

3 tsp chilli oil
2 tsp Chinese black vinegar (or use balsamic)
2 tsp sugar
1 tbsp soy sauce
1 tbsp sesame oil
2 tbsp sesame paste (or to taste)
2–3 tbsp water
1 tsp Sichuan peppercorns, toasted, or dry fried, ground and sieved (only if the sauce is served with chicken)

First mix together the chilli oil, vinegar, sugar and sesame oil; stirring until the sugar is dissolved. Use chopsticks to stir in the sesame paste, then gradually add the water, stopping when the sauce has reached the consistency you desire. Lastly, if the sauce is for chicken, add the Sichuan peppercorns.

small amounts of the controlling flavour. Thus, if a dish is too sour, something spicy might make it appetizing (Thai cooks add chilli to grapefruit and other underripe fruits); too bitter, add salt (this is how we make many greens palatable), and too sweet add something sour (a well appreciated combination). A touch of bitterness can offset spiciness in a dish, though, failing that, sweet, the creator of pungent, also works well. And a sweet flavour can do wonders to mask an excess of salt. One

Sour:
vinegar • lemon juice • tamarind • olives

Sweet (naturally sweet ingredients which have an harmonizing action):
honey • palm sugar • liquorice • rock sugar • coconut

Bitter:
vinegar • cocoa powder • wine (slightly bitter) • tangerine lemon and grapefruit peel • turmeric, fenugreek and some other indian spices

Pungent:
ginger • onions, • garlic • chilies and Sichuan peppercorns • mustard • black pepper • most herbs and spices commonly used in the West

Salty:
oyster sauce (salty and sweet) • sea vegetables • soy sauce, • rock salt • sea salt • dried or pickled vegetables • fermented bean pastes

(See previous chapter for the flavours of common meats, fruits and vegetables).

酸甜苦辣咸

of the most popular dishes that we taught in my cooking school was *guai wei'r ji* ('strange-flavoured' chicken), where shreds of tender chicken meat are topped with a sesame paste sauce, which is sweet, sour, spicy and salty. There was one occasion when the lid fell off the soy sauce bottle and the sauce was frighteningly salty. Xiao Ding did not panic – instead she added more sugar and the taste was, thankfully, masked. Sadly, this practice has been adopted by food manufacturers who use salt as a preservative in sweet products and create overprocessed versions of flavour combinations which at first appear satisfying but leave the body feeling cheated. Lemon or blueberry muffins taste good because they are sweet and sour, but the large amount of sugar used in commercial recipes also hides incredibly high levels of salt. Cheating nature in this way will not result in a well-balanced body; the equivalent Chinese meal would be a bowl of *zhou* with splash of soy or fish sauce (salty) and another of chilli sauce (pungent and sweet).

Xing – *shape*

Vital as balancing the flavours is, this is not the only weapon in the Chinese cook's armoury. When choosing his ingredients a Chinese chef will not only be aware of what will taste good, or can be made to taste good, but also what looks good. Shape can be an intrinsic quality of an ingredient – as with long thin beansprouts, the knobbly heads of cauliflower and or pieces of sweetcorn – or it can be fashioned by the chef to allow an ingredient to cook in a certain way. Over the years, as I picked crisp slivers of carrot or perfectly fashioned pieces of broccoli from colourful stir-fries, tossed wafer-thin slices of meat and vegetables into a simmering pot or delved into clay bowls with my chopsticks to find perfect squares of beancurd, I began to appreciate that the shape of ingredients affects both their appearance and eating quality. Pieces that are all the same size cook evenly and maintain their shape through the cooking process, resulting in a dish that is appetizing

Slicing and dicing

By now you will appreciate that most of the hard work in Chinese cooking is in the preparation. An invaluable tool for the Chinese chef is his *dao* (the word means 'knife' but in the West we usually describe these large, flat, rectangular blades as 'choppers'), used for practically every cutting or shaping task, and for mashing, mincing and scooping up cut ingredients too.

A set of sharp knives can do many of the same jobs as the chopper but would not be in keeping with the simplicity of the Chinese kitchen, and no single other knife is as versatile as a *dao* – nor can they be wielded at such speed or used for mashing and scooping functions. Anyone can use a chopper – and practically everyone in China does. It is simply a question of practice. There are three rules for use: sharp, straight and concentrate.

A brief run-through of the Chinese vocabulary of food shapes may help you think about how you can make your meals more visually interesting but uniform:

Da kuai'r – chunks. Large chunks are used for stewing or braising. Chicken and other fowl are chopped bones and all, so as to make a rich and nutritious stock, to which fresh or dried vegetables or beancurd are added.

大块

Qie pian'r – slices. Long round vegetables are best for slicing. Use the chopper to cut a slice off one side to create a flat surface, then lay the vegetable horizontally and slice. Slices are best lightly simmered, or shallow, or deep-fried, since stir-frying tends to break up the pieces.

切片

Si – slivers. Shredded or matchstick pieces are ideal for cooking quickly over a high heat and are also used in steamed dishes. First cut the vegetable into long slices (you can achieve minimum waste if you slice on the diagonal). Then with one hand flatten out the slices and in the other use the *dao* to shred them.

丝

小条 *Tiao* – small strips. Only choice cuts of meat or tender, firm beancurd are suitable for cutting into finger-sized pieces for stir-frying. These pieces are often partnered with lengths of vegetable (see *duan* below).

段 *Duan* – lengths. Ingredients that are long and thin, such as green beans or celery, can simply be chopped into lengths, often on the diagonal for a more attractive appearance. They are usually blanched before stir-frying.

丁 *Ding* – diced. Firm vegetables such as potato, bamboo shoots, carrot and water chestnut and lean pieces of chicken, pork, beancurd and fish are all suitable for cutting into small cubes. First cut into thick slices, then chop into strips and then into cubes. These cubes can be cooked together with naturally small foods such as pinenuts, peanuts, peas or sweetcorn.

剁碎 *Duo sui* – minced. Chinese chefs mince food with a chopper, may use your electric mixer. Minced meats, vegetables and beancurd are used as a stuffing, or sometimes quickly fried and sprinkled over a dish.

大致 **剁碎** *Da zhi duo sui* – roughly minced. Garlic, ginger, spring onion, chilies and other supporting ingredients are cut into tiny pieces for a variety of uses.

and an eating experience that is strangely more satisfying than when foods have been randomly chopped.

Having become used to eating and preparing dishes where the ingredients are uniformly fashioned into a particular shape I find myself surprisingly offended if presented, for instance, with a minestrone soup where large irregular lumps of potato take their place among long slivers of cabbage, and round slices of carrot. Such a meal neither looks as good nor is as enjoyable to eat as when the same ingredients are cut into pieces of the same size.

Se – *colour*

The vibrant colours of the Chinese market are reflected in the Chinese table. I particularly love the way many market stallholders sell only one type of ingredient, so the tomato stall will be a sea of red, verdant greens represent every shade of the colour and piles of silver bean and yellow soy sprouts glint in the sunlight. Other stalls display a colourful mosaic, laid with much thought so that brightly coloured carrots or sweetcorn and my favourite red radish provide light relief among the greens and browns.

It is not difficult, therefore, for the chef to bring home the foods he needs to create a meal that is equally attractive to the eye. The homely stir-fry of tomato and egg that graces many a family table is a significant dish for its use of contrasting colours as well as a nutritious combination. The tiny flecks of carrot in a pale green winter melon soup catch the eye as well as representing the *yin* and the *yang*, opposing forces that always contain a little of each other.

Kou gan – *texture*

It is easy to appreciate the attractive appearance and vivid colour combinations of a Chinese meal. The final dimension,

Tomato and egg
Ji dan chao xi hong shi

鸡
蛋
炒
西
红
柿

This simple homely dish will add colour to any multi-dish table, but is also a good choice for breakfast or a light lunch.

3 tomatoes

2 eggs

½ tsp finely chopped ginger

½ tsp finely chopped spring onion

1 tsp sugar

½ tsp salt (or to taste)

1 tbsp oil

½ tsp sesame oil

First peel the tomatoes by putting them into a heat-proof bowl, pouring boiling water over them and waiting a few minutes. The skins should now slip off easily. Remove the core and chop roughly.

Beat the eggs and season with a small pinch of salt.

Heat the wok to medium to high heat. Add half the oil, turn the heat down to medium and tip in the beaten egg. As it hits the oil it will puff up; stir it with a spatula to break it into pieces, then remove and set aside.

Clean the wok, heat again, add the rest of the oil, turn down the heat and add the ginger, spring onion and tomatoes. Cook quickly (all you need to do is warm the mixture through), then add the sugar and salt. Mix in well and return the eggs to the pan.

Stir again to mix together the eggs and tomato. Turn off the heat and finish with a splash of sesame oil.

texture or *kou gan* (which literally means 'mouth feel') takes a bit more getting used to. Nowadays one of my favourite dishes is called *Lo Han Zhai* ('Buddha's Delight'), but I have to admit that it took a while for me to get used to it. It is renowned for its esoteric ingredients, which include bamboo shoots and beansprouts (both crunchy), silver ear-fungus (slippery and chewy) and a sea vegetable best translated as 'hair moss' (hair is exactly what it looks like and feels like in the mouth). My ultimate *kou gan* experience, though, is something called *zhu ti*, which is the pith of the bamboo stalk, found between the outer and inner layers. The first time I found it I was convinced it was from some aquatic creature, or possibly an old gauze dressing off somebody's toe! *Zhu ti* is actually a terrific ingredient because it absorbs the flavours of whatever else is in the soup and releases them slowly into the mouth, resulting again in the comfortable feeling of satiety that I associate with Chinese food.

If you start to take texture into consideration you can lift your cooking to new levels. Chinese chefs often add pinenuts to sweetcorn – the eye doesn't even see them half the time, but they provide a great treat for the mouth (and they are full of healthy oils, too). Minced water chestnuts add a bite to pork or tofu balls; bamboo shoots, lotus root and mushrooms provide a contrast in a stew and are even used in fried rice; a handful of beansprouts makes a unusual crunchy filling for a creamy omelette. The mix of textures can be within the meal as well as in the individual dishes: make your vegetables into purées, steam a whole fish or chicken over a very low heat until the flesh melts in the mouth. Chinese chefs use a wealth of dried vegetables to add interest: you can try sun-dried tomatoes, strips of seaweed or reconstituted fungus.

A basic Chinese store-cupboard

The following bottled seasonings are all mentioned in the text and will enable you to cook most of the recipes in this book or add interest to your own creations.

Chinese cooking wine *(liao jiu)*: This brings out the flavour *(ti wei'r)*. It is used for pre-treating practically all meats and fish before cooking and also sprinkled on stir-fries and splashed into stews. The most famous cooking wine is from Shao Xing, but any rice wine can be used.

Vinegar *(cu)*: This is much more heavily used in Chinese cooking than it is in the West. It is believed to dispel the rankness *(xin wei'r)* of meat or fish, but also adds a depth of flavour and contrast to cold mixed and stir-fried dishes. The mild-flavoured, rice vinegar is the most commonly used. Dark, black vinegars, fermented from sorghum, are popular in the north of China and are used as a dip for dumplings.

Soy sauce *(jiang you)*: This is easier to use than salt, and as well as being salty *(xian)* it adds colour and additional liquid to cooked dishes or dressings. There are two types of soy sauce in common usage: *sheng chou*, (literally translated 'young' and sold in the West as 'light'); and *lao chou* ('old sauce') – called 'dark' in the West. The light soy sauce has the fresher and stronger taste and is used for dressing cold dishes and some stir-fries. Dark soy sauce offers no taste advantage but is used for heavy stews, some beef and lamb dishes and whenever a deep colour is required.

Sesame oil *(xiang you)*: This should not be used for cooking because it does not hold the heat, but it can be splashed onto hot and cold dishes and soups to add or enhance the *xiang*, or fragrant taste.

A note about MSG: Monosodium glutamate (MSG) is a flavour enhancer used by some Chinese restaurants. It is a chemical that occurs naturally in some foods, including Parmesan cheese, Shitake mushrooms and seaweed, from which it was originally extracted. It was first imported into China from Japan in the early 1900s and welcomed by chefs trying to make *cai* taste good when fresh ingredients were scarce. MSG is colourless and flavourless but stimulates the nerve endings on the tongue, thus enhancing the eating experience. Unfortunately, this means that it can also stimulate other nerves, causing headaches and twitching. It is not a traditional Chinese food. I have never used it in my cooking school and it is not used in high quality restaurants. You do *not* need it in your store cupboard.

Time to cook

Despite the ease with which the Chinese chef works, no two, or three, ingredients are ever thrown together without consideration. A Chinese chef would never slap a piece of steak in a frying pan or boil potatoes whole. A piece of beef might be treated with wine and cooked with a range of seasonings such as ginger, spring onion and salt and possibly much stronger flavours (in western China, chilies, and in the south, oyster sauce) then partnered with tomatoes or slivers of carrot. Potatoes are generally shredded and stir-fried with Sichuan peppercorns or dried chilies – but I love them sliced and braised with fresh green chilli and soy sauce.

For the uninitiated to reach the degree of food knowledge of the average Chinese domestic cook is long-term ambition, and cultural differences may mean that it is impossible fully to appreciate all the aspects of the Chinese diet. But you can begin to think more about how you prepare, season and cook your ingredients. All that chopping may seem a bit daunting, especially when followed by a hot wok session. But look back to Chapters Five and Six and remember to base your richer and tastier stir-fried dishes with lighter soups, stews and simmered dishes, which are very simple to prepare and do not require last-minute attention.

The aim of this chapter is to encourage you to make dishes that always taste, look and feel good and to move away from the idea that there are two types of food: the nice rich fattening ones, which you want to eat but shouldn't, and the low-fat, tasteless boring ones which you don't want to eat, but should. In China richer heavier dishes grace the same table as delicate and light ones, but there is no trade-off – they are all enjoyed for their various characteristics.

Of course, it is one thing to enjoy sweet-and-sour aubergine or to appreciate the fragrance of a fresh wok-cooked fish if you have been brought up on such a diet, but if you hanker after steak and chips, pasta with creamy, rich sauces, or cakes and biscuits and luscious puddings, are they really a substitute?

In the first instance just try to incorporate the Chinese approach to cooking into your meal plans. This does not necessarily entail your giving up your household favourites; what you should be focusing on is adding to and developing your diet and eating more and different foods at every opportunity.

nine

Choose 'live' over 'dead' or processed foods

九

'Consider how much time and effort have been spent before food is ready for consumption: in farming, harvesting, processing and cooking, not to mention the slaughtering of animal lives — all this to please our palate.'

HUANG TING JIAN (AD 1050–1110)

Qi, life-force, is all around us, in the earth, in the air and in the heavens. It is found in the balance of *yin* and *yang* and in the flow of the Five Elements cycle. When we are young our supply of *Qi* is plentiful, though all too often we abuse it and suffer in later life. As we get older our supply of *Qi* gradually diminishes, until we become weak and eventually die.

A curious incident one October evening helped me to understand the real importance of *Qi* in the Chinese diet. It was the end of the October National Day holiday and we had just returned from a weekend at Beidaihe, Beijing's nearest beach resort and favourite summertime retreat of Communist

Party officials. With the new motorway, the drive was only two hours and, having left after a fine lunch of fresh sea food, we arrived home in good time for the children to get ready for school and for me to prepare the evening meal. Leaving our bags in an untidy heap just inside the front door, I went into the kitchen to check out the fridge – but I never got that far. The room was alive with little white maggots. I screamed for help, wondering whether crying was an option, and noticed with horror that the worms had two beady little eyes and a black nose.

Tim started to suck them up into the vacuum cleaner and Max and Christian suddenly remembered urgent engagements with their friends in other compounds, so I attacked the cupboards. I found infestations in my black sesame seeds, walnuts, pinenuts, almonds, Chinese dates and wolfberries. The 'Job's tears' were crawling as was a bag full of dried aubergine slices. We had recently taken a trip to the countryside where, in my usual spirit of culinary adventure, I had stocked up on local produce. The original infestation could probably be traced back to one, or several, of these purchases of dried fruits and vegetables, nuts and seeds. Because I had bought so much I had left them all in the flimsy plastic bags they came in, rather than taking the precaution of transferring them to airtight containers.

At first I thought that the untouched wheat biscuits, branflakes, the extruded wheat squares and even the crunchy wheat and malted barley nuggets had been protected from infestation by the packaging: my 'healthy' breakfast cereals had all been imported from Australia at great expense. But although all the packets had been opened – in fact most them were gaping – they were all bug free. A half-empty box of salted crackers left over from some party was also untouched, as was an open packet of digestive biscuits that should have been in a tin but weren't. As the contents of my kitchen cupboard were spread over tables and sideboards the pattern was unmistakable. The maggots preferred brown rice to white, and buckwheat or wholewheat flour to bleached. The connection was clear: creepy crawlies are not slaves to their taste buds, the pressures of advertising or convenience. Nature directs them to the foods that will provide the most nourishment – live, not processed, foods.

The following morning I tipped out the contents of the breakfast cereals into bowls amid screams of 'maggot hunt!' 'Don't worry, the maggots know better than to eat these pieces of sugared cardboard,' I told the kids triumphantly. 'Enjoy what's left because I'm not buying them again.'

Live food is better than dead

After the creepy crawly incident, 'live food is better than dead' became the new motto in our household. Real food does not come from supermarkets, or even from factories. It grows; it lives. All life forms contain Qi. Our bodies are living organisms; it is better to nurture them with live foods if we can. Qi is sometimes translated as 'energy', which leads to a comparison with the western concept of calories. This is totally misleading. Qi is not about quantity, it is about quality: and quality is what the Chinese cuisine is all about.

Once you acknowledge the concept of Qi in food, you will truly understand the need to eat a diet made up of fresh, natural foods and have the confidence to refute the health claims that food manufacturers make about hundreds of processed and packaged goods.

The main characteristic of Qi is motion or the activity of life. When a food goes bad or rancid or grows mould, these are all indication that Qi is present. Absence of activity tends to mean that Qi is either suspended or absent. Hence preserving may compromise Qi, but some modern processing methods that allow foods to be stored for extensive periods destroy it completely.

Where Qi is suspended it can re-activate to some degree when the food is released from its preserved state. Tinned tomatoes, once exposed to the air, soon grow mould; pickled onions will eventually decay once unsealed and opened. Small amounts of bottled or canned foods, using naturally available preservatives such as salt and sugar, can make a contribution to a balanced diet, both Chinese or western, and there are circumstances where these add variety to a regime that would otherwise be very limited. Freezing is another method that nature has made available. A Chinese friend once told me that her family would always kill their pig at Chinese New Year (in late January or early February) and then make a massive pork stew. After the holiday the remainder would be left in the central courtyard to freeze; when the family 'felt like eating meat', they would hack off a chunk, heat it, adding cellophane noodles and chopped white cabbage before serving.

In China natural methods are used to preserve foods, which are then used to enhance, not replace, a natural food diet. Some traditional processing methods can increase the nutrient value of foods. For example, many of the fermented pastes used in Chinese cooking have been found to contain vitamin B12, a nutrient many people lack. Additionally many of these products are a source of probiotics that can enhance the 'good' bacteria in the gut and are increasingly thought to have many health benefits. Bamboo shoots, a source of silica, are preserved in salt water in the north of China, and is available all year round.

The basis of the Chinese diet is freshly picked, freshly prepared foods. In China most people are still close to their food source. I was reminded of this every time we visited the home of the cheery Guo Gui Lan. By covering the distance of a medium sized London commute (less than an hour's drive) we entered another world, a world the Chinese call *nong cun* (peasant village) where extended families live off their neatly arranged smallholdings, and signs painted on redbrick walls encourage the population to 'grow crops not children'.

Guo Gui Lan's piercing black eyes danced out of her weather-beaten face and she smiled continually, setting wrinkles into her paper-thin skin. Like many Chinese people I met she seemed oblivious to the temperature and always wore the same tweed jacket that only just met around her stout torso. While appearing unaffected by Beijing's new prosperity, Guo Gui Lan knew how to take advantage of it. As well as running a roadside restaurant for people en route to the well-known Black Dragon Pool further up the road, Guo Gui Lan rented out rooms in the spacious peasant-style courtyard house which she shared with her diffident husband, whose name we never did learn, her son and daughter-in-law and a collection of motley dogs, some chickens and a pig.

Guo Gui Lan would always make it clear what she would prefer us to order from her seemingly extensive menu. On one occasion when she had convinced us that we really wanted fish, I wandered out towards the brick-built loo and found her dabbling around with a net in what looked like a drain just between the restaurant and the road. I wasn't too worried, as I knew that wherever the drain went, it wasn't connected to the loo – which was just a hole in the ground. But I was sufficiently curious to peer down the hole on my way back and saw that the water looked clean and fast flowing. I never did work out if the fish had swum up into it from the reservoir or if it had been put there earlier in the day, but it arrived flapping vigorously; no self-respecting Chinese chef would choose a fish that had been sitting around over one that had just been caught and dispatched. Later, lightly seasoned with ginger and spring onion, it simply melted in the mouth; everyone said it was delicious, and I said nothing.

The highlights of meals at Guo Gui Lan's were always the vegetables. I loved to see what *ye cai* ('wild vegetables') were in season that month, and whether she would stir-fry them or serve then cold, lightly dressed with garlic and vinegar and a touch of sesame oil. Once she proudly showed us some chilies she had just harvested, asking if we liked them. 'Oh yes!' we cried enthusiastically, unaware that they were to be the main, if not the only ingredient of the finished dish. It was a dish that was surprisingly edible as the chilies, lightly stewed and tempered with sugar and vinegar, were pungent and flavoursome rather than 'blow your head off' hot.

The chilies that Guo Gui Lan did not manage to push on to unsuspecting visitors would be hung up to dry in the sun for use throughout the winter. At different times of year all manner of other delicacies would be laid out in the sunshine: strips of radish, greens, fungus, aubergines, soya beans and even bright orange persimmon. Drying is a natural process that accords with the Five-Element cycle: *fire* is used to dry plants (*wood*) which are then revived by *water*. Dried foods, like the fermented and salted ingredients mentioned earlier, play an important role in enhancing Chinese cuisine, and often add interesting textures to dishes. Many great western recipes are also dependent on dried ingredients such as herbs, olives, capers and sun-dried tomatoes, and these are worthy members of your store cupboard.

Drying foods appears not to compromise *Qi* significantly, as my maggots were quick to recognize. Consumption of fresh food by animals, or humans for that matter, is also representative of the *fire* stage in the Five Elements cycle: the digestive system burns food which is eventually excreted and returned to the earth.

Traditional preserving methods all use nature's resources; modern processing and preserving practices do not. Extremes of temperature adulterate foods to the extent that the activity of the Five Elements cycle is halted altogether. Take the processing of oil, which has recently been the subject of much publicity. Food scientists were thrilled to discover that by heating it to very high temperatures and hydrogenating, or partially hydrogenating it, they could prolong its shelf life almost indefinitely, thus producing all sorts of delicious treats. The problem is that that hydrogenating oils changes their structure so that they are are damaging, if not dangerous, to health.[9] To the Chinese mind it is completely obvious that heating oil to the temperatures needed to hydrogenate it would destroy its *Qi* and make it inaccessible to the body. The first naturally pressed oils, which command a premium price and are now being heralded as total panaceas, are the same products that Chinese peasants have been producing for generations.

Qi *is everywhere in the natural world*

The moment we take a food from its natural environment we interfere with nature's *Qi* flow. In an ideal world we would eat all our food on the day it is picked, since the further a foodstuff is removed from its source the weaker its supply of *Qi*. There is *Qi* in soil (Earth) that has been nurtured by traditional farming methods. In China crops are rotated and the nation's major crop, the soya bean, transfers nitrogen back into the soil, ensuring that the earth remains fertile.

Have you ever noticed how carrots or potatoes last much longer if you store them without washing them? The connection with the soil helps to maintain their *Qi*. Modern nutritionists acknowledge that the vitamin content of most vegetables decreases with storage and decry the loss of many minerals that used to find their way into the diet through the soil on vegetables. My grandfather always said, 'You need to eat a peck of dirt before you die.'

Malnutrition in the midst of plenty

We spurn nutritious food such as offal, seaweed and some fungus without trying to make them palatable because they aren't attractive to the eye. We eat all manner of adulterated foodstuffs instead – foods that provide plenty of calories and adequate amounts of proteins, cabohydrates and fats, but few, if any, of the micro-nutrients that modern nutritionists are beginning to recognize as necessary in order to make our bodies function well. While we have been able to trick our senses into believing that these manufactured and artificial foodstuffs are an acceptable substitute for the real thing in the short term, the western world is now suffering from malnutrition in the midst of plenty.[10]

Take the 'healthy' breakfast cereals that my maggots were so unimpressed with. Cereal-makers create a slurry of grains, put them into an extruder and then force them out of a little hole at high pressure. In *Fighting the Food Giants*, Paul Stitt tells us how the extrusion process destroys most of the nutri-ents in the grains. Yet packaged and processed foods, even those low in nutrients, seem to offer a security that many people find it difficult to walk away from. Food manufacturers take advantage of our lack of connection with the source of our food by offering us calorie counts and nutritional breakdowns – but these are just smokescreens. While low-fat versions of your favourite treats may contain fewer calories, to call this a 'health benefit' is a misnomer.

In traditional societies pickled meats and vegetables, jams and chutneys contained salt and sugar in order to add variety to a diet that might otherwise have been very limited. Unfortunately, though, the human body has a natural affinity for these flavours through their relationship with the spleen/stomach (salty is associated with the earth element and sweet is the flavour that enters it), and the spleen/stomach's association with the mouth. Since the advent of mass produc-tion this predilection has become disastrous.

The word is out of course, and manufacturers are now having a field day finding new ways to make their processed products 'healthier'. Modern nutritionists have made great strides in recent years in identifying the roles of essential fatty acids, anti-oxidants and many previously-unacknowledged micronutrients. Ever more nutritional claims are finding their way onto colourful cartons and shiny wrappers which once boasted only about protein, calcium and vitamin content. All this noise diverts consumers from the fact that these newly discovered health-giving substances are all first derived and best consumed from natural foods, which is what the Chinese principles of the *Qi* and the Five Elements/Five Flavours have always made clear.

If you can trust nature to provide you with the nourishment that that your body needs, and learn to make less obviously palatable foods into tasty dishes, your body will be much healthier. If you have to eat processed or prepared food, take it for what it is – a food substitute, not real food and certainly not a meal.

Real food

Eating in China is all about real food. Nature has endowed us with the whole spectrum of food types and the ability to make these more digestible and palatable. The Five Elements that make up the natural world from a Taoist viewpoint can all be represented by different types of vegetables and fruits: *wood* foods are green, especially those which grow upwards and have branches, so persevere with that broccoli when the kids are young; and try asparagus spears too. Brightly coloured fire fruits and vegetables often grow round bunches of seeds: spicy chilies and red peppers, pumpkin and butternut squash, but sometimes have a central stone, as with cherries, mangoes, peaches and plums. The *earth* vegetables, sweet potatoes, carrots, swede, celeriac and potatoes, grow in the ground and are more subdued in colour; while *earth* fruits, apples and pears, are dense and tightly packed. *Metal's* fruits and vegetables hide their properties, so need to be peeled before eating: these include citrus fruits and bananas, ginger, radishes, garlic and onions. Easily overlooked, *water* foods include sea vegetables and those grown in damp conditions, including watercress, mushrooms and other fungi.

The question of meat

You will have noticed that the above list makes no mention of meat. We could categorize flesh foods according to the

Five-Element concept, too — animals that eat plants (*wood*), those that eat fruits, those that live in the *water* — but you will notice that they are all one step removed. Meat, in its own way, provides mankind with the ultimate 'convenience food'. Plants absorb the sun's energy through their leaves and construct energy through photosynthesis. Animals eat those plants. As omnivores, we can obtain our nutrients directly through eating many different plants, or indirectly, 'second hand', through the flesh of a small number of animals species.

Chinese Buddhists believe that the *Qi* we get from eating plants is superior to the *Qi* we obtain from the flesh of dead animals: the former is known as *primary Qi*, the latter is considered *secondary*.

Chinese people do eat meat, and you will see that it has its place in the Five-Flavours chart, with seafoods and some organ meats having particular value as they offer natural sources of the *salty* and *bitter* flavours. But throughout this book I have stressed how a good Chinese diet includes meat in moderation. The Chinese character for a house or home is *jia*, which derives from a pictogram of a pig under a roof. It was only after I had spent some time in the country that this apparent insult to the native population made sense. 'Pigs', Guo Gui Lan explained, 'eat all the waste that cannot be disposed of elsewhere and when their time is up, we eat all of them.' I decided not to think too hard about what she meant exactly by 'all the waste' or even 'all of them' and focused instead on the environmental advantages of this age-old system. Like all smallholders Guo Gui Lan would kill only one pig a year, which meant that meat was used very sparingly in her recipes. If I took visitors to her who I knew would feel unsatisfied without their daily dose of animal protein, I would put in a request in advance and she would manage to find an old chicken to throw in the pot. Guo Gui Lan's annual pig would not last long in the West, where we rely heavily on meat as a centrepiece to meals, but pork in particular, because of its ecological and economic advantages, has an accepted place in the overall diet in China. When Chinese people say *rou* (meat), they are always referring to pork. Other meats that feature even less commonly in the everyday diet are referred to by species: *ji rou* (chicken), *niu rou* (beef), *ya rou* (duck), and they are all believed to make a contribution to good health if eaten as what Chinese food therapy describes as a 'tonic', or a particularly nourishing food. Tonics are usually taken when the body is exhausted or recovering from illness. Small amounts of mutton or duck might be stewed with onion or star anise to boost deficient *yang*, or beef might be eaten to nourish the *Qi* and blood.

The vegetarian movement is not big in China, except among Buddhist monks; meat consumption has never been sufficiently significant to warrant giving it up. In *The China Study*, Dr Campbell recommends a vegetarian diet as a result of his findings about the link between excessive consumption of animal protein and the prevalent diseases of the western world.

In America, about 15 per cent of total calorie intake comes from proteins and 80 per cent of that is from animal-based products, whereas in rural China less than 10 per cent of total calories come from protein, only ten per cent of which is from animal-based foods.[11] Two observations from *The China Study* are sufficient to illustrate that the lack of animal protein in the Chinese diet is not detrimental to health. On the contrary:

At the time of our study, the death rate from coronary heart disease was seventeen times higher among American men than rural Chinese men.

(*The China Study*, p.79)

The American death rate from breast cancer was five times higher than the rural Chinese rate.

(*The China Study*, p.79)

Dr Campbell's study shows that the environment created in the body by a diet high in animal protein is conducive to the spread of cancerous cells. Protein from soya beans, on the other hand, brings the protection of no less than six compounds believed to protect against cancer,[12] including isoflavones, which have had a lot of publicity for their ability to block the type of oestrogen hormone implicated in increased breast cancer levels.

Soya – the vegetable plus

I have heard it said that if China had not cultivated soya beans – which are not only a complete protein source containing all of the eight essential amino acids but also of benefit to other crops – it would never have been able to feed its people. (Though the flip-side of this argument is that if China had focused on animal protein, the population would never have grown so large in the first place.) Chinese peasant-farmers were not only clever to grow what has now been recognized as one of the most nutritious foods in the world, but they also found a way to make it into a product which was more easily digestible than the bean itself and capable of infinite variety of uses – beancurd.

The Chinese name for soya bean is *huang dou*, meaning yellow bean, but the generic word *dou* (bean) is often used to describe soya beans. Beancurd, or *dou fu*, (which literally means fermented beans, originated in China), although it is better known in the West by its Japanese name, *tofu*. When I first started working with it I had a tendency to use both *dou fu* and *tofu* interchangeably, which confused many a student, so, for the sake of clarity, I have taken to using the literal English name, beancurd.

Unlike many foreigners, I never had a problem with beancurd's soft and slightly slimy texture. Sometimes I wonder if I was born on the wrong side of the world: my mother had to force-feed me custard as a child, and I still have bad dreams about the time I found skin in my grandmother's milk jelly. Indoctrinated as I was by the idea that the calcium in dairy products was essential for healthy bones, I persevered and grew to enjoy cheese even though I never felt completely comfortable after eating it. Only after I arrived in China and discovered a nation that appeared to be thriving on a dairy-free diet did I entertain the idea that there might be an alternative.

It is now known that calcium can be absorbed to build bones only if other factors are also present, including many vitamins (especially vitamin K) and minerals (especially magnesium).[13] So drinking quantities of milk will not benefit the body in the same way as, say, using small amounts of cheese or yogurt in a vegetable dish. Even better, you could create a dish out of beancurd, a natural source of both vitamin K and magnesium, and serve it with a host of other vegetables.

In China, beancurd is usually made by cottage industries that work through the night to be ready for the early morning markets. The process involves soaking the soya beans, grinding them to a pulp with water, extracting the liquid soya milk, boiling it, then using a setting agent, either salt, lemon juice or, now more commonly, gypsum.

Most beancurd is sold in blocks, varing in texture according to how much water has been pressed out during the setting process. There are two main types: firm, which is often lightly smoked, and soft, which is also known as 'silken' beancurd. Soft or silken beancurd is generally used for cold dishes, often simply topped with minced spring onion, coriander, salt and sesame oil, or diced in soups. The firm varieties lend themselves better to deep or shallow frying. Most chefs prepare a *jiachang* ('home-taste') dish, which varies according to the local ingredients available but is always rich and flavoursome. Then there are a host of other types to choose from too: pressed shapes, sheets, shreds and beancurd skin, to name but a few. These might be flavoured with five-spice or even pig's blood, or sold plain, ready to absorb whatever seasonings are used in a recipe.

Most western supermarkets and many speciality stores now offer a firm and a soft variety, the latter is sometimes sold as 'silken'. Unfortunately, unfamiliarity with the product sometimes leads to incorrect labelling: I have found some of the long-life 'firm' types still too soft to use for frying or stews. A firm beancurd will not crumble when cut or fall apart when simmered, so it is perfect for use in stews or stir-fries or even roasted; when mashed it can be used in terrine-type dishes. Soft or silken beancurd, on the other hand, is not very suitable for cooking. In China it is eaten cold, either sliced or crumbled and dressed, and used to stuff vegetables. It works in shakes and smoothies too.

If you are not convinced about beancurd, don't close this book with a sigh and conclude that this way of eating is not

Pan-fried beancurd
Guo ta dou fu

There are many versions of this simple dish: sometimes the pieces are bound together in an egg pancake, sometimes they are served with a light sauce. I prefer to serve them as individual pieces, which we eat for breakfast dipped in sweet chilli sauce.

锅
塌
豆
腐

300 g/10 oz/2 cups block of firm beancurd
1 tsp finely chopped spring onion
1 tsp finely chopped ginger
1 tsp Chinese cooking wine
small dish of cornflour (for dipping)
1 beaten egg
½ tsp salt (or to taste)
1 tbsp oil

This recipe is best made in a large flat-bottomed frying pan rather than a wok. Slice the beancurd block into pieces of about ½ cm thick. Sprinkle the pieces with the Chinese cooking wine, and then dip them first in the cornflour and then in the egg.

Heat the frying pan to a medium heat and sprinkle the salt over the bottom (this stops the pieces sticking as well as seasoning the dish); add the oil. When the oil is hot place the beancurd squares in the frying pan, fry for about a minute, until the pieces can be easily lifted, then flip them over.

Sprinkle the cooked side of the beancurd with a little chopped ginger and spring onion and flip over again. Add the rest of the ginger and spring onion to the other side, then fry both sides until they are golden brown.

Serve immediately.

for you. It took me ten years to reach the stage when I am excited to have a slab in my fridge, and I did not have to overcome an initial dislike. My own family's experience shows me that preference for one food over another is more to do with situation and habit than with genetic predisposition. In my cooking classes, many of my female students blamed their reluctance to experiment on their husbands' 'real-men-don't-eat-tofu' mentality; but I was pretty certain that those same students had no idea how to cook it and that the recalcitrant men in their lives had not tried it tossed in mouth-numbing Sichuan pepper sauce or lightly dusted in cornflour and deep fried, served up with a spicy dip. The first dish I learnt to cook with confidence was *Guo ta dou fu* (pan-fried beancurd, see recipe p.144), which I jokingly describe as Chinese 'eggy bread'. It is delicious served with a sweet chilli sauce:

Having had the opportunity to observe the Chinese diet first hand over a ten-year period, I believe that Chinese food culture is so nutritious and healthy not only because of the minor role played by meat, but also because of what Chinese people eat instead of meat. There are very few health benefits of a vegetarian diet which is made up of processed bread and potatoes, or even cheese, eggs, bread and potatoes. The gaping hole that appears when we take meat out of our western diet, or even minimize it, needs to be filled with plant-based foods. They are all out there in nature: in the soil, on the ground, in bushes and trees, even in the water, and there are plenty of seasonings available to make them into tasty nutritious meals.

The Chinese have managed to find a middle road, which is their way. But if you have been at one extreme it may be necessary to go to the other before finding the centre. Teenagers, in the *fire* stage of their lives, are quick to make decisions and to embrace change. One hot Friday night in 2004, my son Christian, then aged thirteen, arrived home from his school trip to Mongolia. He had had the time of his life in the Gobi Desert, riding on a camel singing 'I'm just a teenage dirtbag baby' at the top of his voice. After dancing on the Shrine of the Great Sheep and climbing the Sand-dune of the Singing Sand Gorge, the group had visited a Buddhist temple and shared the monks' vegetarian lunch. Whether it was the monks who influenced him ultimately or the new good-looking redhead from Scotland I never found out, but he announced firmly that he had given up eating meat.

Some teenagers wear black from head to toe, others pierce their tongues; I reckoned a bout of vegetarianism was pretty harmless. And it wasn't as if I needed to revise my style of cooking completely, since our diet had been based for some time on the idea that 'the vegetables are the dishes'. In fact I found that having to prepare meals without any meat at all made me far more adventurous as a cook. Vegetarians can eat amazingly well on a selection of Chinese *cai*, though I also started to look to other culinary traditions, particularly from India and the Middle East for more substantial 'one pot' dishes. I experimented with curries and kormas, tagines and tabboulehs, and noticed how I could still manage to achieve a balance of flavours and a range of cooking methods with different cuisines and, of course, round off the meal with a large bowl of a staple food, such as rice, couscous, barley or bulgar wheat.

Those countries with the strongest culinary traditions are those that have not lost touch with their peasant origins. And there is no way that the homely dishes eaten in country homes feature large chunks of animal protein. Indian food is an example. No doubt your local take-away will offer vindaloos, madras and kormas, made with beef, lamb or chicken, and then list a few vegetable 'side dishes' at the end of the menu. Yet Indian vegetarian cuisine is one of the most substantial and creative. Think about it: when you enjoy a Chicken Madras, is it the spices and seasonings that make the dish, or the lumps of flesh? Influenced by China, I have managed to adopt a 'middle way' approach in our household and my cooking, continuing to use small amounts of organic or free-range meat from time to time for those who prefer a carnivorous option, simmering an organic chicken occasionally and using the stock for noodles. More and more, though, I find that the vegetable option is the one preferred.

As ever, I urge you to consider alternatives and expand your view of food rather than to embark on a rigorous programme of restriction and denial. Try to incorporate *Qi* in your diet at every opportunity. Primary *Qi* or secondary *Qi*, the choice is yours. Where you may have directed your efforts to reducing your intake of energy in the form of calories you should now consider increasing your intake of real energy or life-force, in the form of *Qi*. As this *Qi* begins to circulate freely in your system you will no longer feel the need to pander to the demands of the mouth and stomach but will want to eat a diet comprised of fresh natural foods.

ten

Respect the body's climate

'The later sages then arose, and men [learned] to take advantage of the origins of fire.'

FROM *LI CHI* (*THE RECORD OF RIGHTS*),
ZHOU DYNASTY TEXT (1027–221 BC)

I once chose a 'house salad' in a small restaurant by the side of a lake in one of Beijing's many parks. The waitress had excitedly proffered a 'western-style' menu, and so as not to disappoint her I chose what appeared to be the safest option, a house salad. Tim opted for the tuna sandwich. When my dish arrived I was horrified to find that, rather than a dish of crunchy greens, I had ordered a mixture of cubed carrot, peas and sweetcorn, tinned peaches and cherries, all bound in a sickly mayonnaise. Tim thought this extremely funny – until he bit into his sandwich, advertised as 'tuna and salad', and found it was full of mashed potato.

'Why don't Chinese people eat salad?' Newcomers to China are quick to notice that while international hotels offer sumptuous salad buffets, these are spurned by the local population. The Chinese have always considered the ability to use fire to cook food as one of the foundations of their civilization and something that separated them from the neighbouring barbarians. By learning to cook food, mankind has been able to expand its diet to include a whole range of plants that might otherwise have been harmful. With new foods come increased nutrients; with increased nutrients comes better health, stronger, fitter bodies and even heightened brain-power. Most grain foods, and many roots and tubers, cannot be easily digested unless cooked, and most civilizations were founded on a carbohydrate of one kind or another.

Yet in modern western societies, raw food is becoming more and more fashionable. Salad is cheap and simple to prepare, so restaurants and supermarket chains can make it readily available. And everyone knows that raw foods have a higher concentration of vitamins than cooked foods – at least recent research points that way. But, what isn't taken into account in the laboratory, is the effort that the body has to make to extract these vitamins. Lightly cooking foods can make their nutrients more easily accessible to the body, so that it can preserve its *Qi* for more important tasks.

Cooking brings the whole Five Element process into play. By taking a piece of broccoli (wood) and, using heat (fire) to boil water in a metal receptacle and adding salt from the earth, we use all Five Elements in order to create a more palatable from of nourishment. Many vegetables are completely indigestible or even toxic when eaten raw; others are just not that kind to the stomach, or not particularly nice to eat. Chinese cooking methods have been refined over the years to ensure that maximum nutrition is extracted from all foodstuffs while making even the most bizarre of ingredients taste good. And of course any nutrients that are leached into cooking water are then drunk in soup.

Cold mixed beancurd stick
Liang ban fu zhu

Dried beancurd sticks (*fu zhu*) are quite readily available in Chinese and Asian supermarkets in the West. Their chewy texture makes them very different from other beancurd products, and those who find regular beancurd too slimy may prefer this variety. They can also be stir-fried or used in braised dishes, but this simple treatment is the most commonly known in Beijing.

凉
拌
腐
竹

100 g/3½ oz/1 cup dried beancurd stick
50 g/¾ oz/½ cup raw peanuts
1 piece star anise
pinch of Sichuan peppercorns
3 sticks celery
1 large carrot (or two small)
2 tsp sesame oil
½–1 tsp salt

Soak the beancurd stick and the peanuts (separately) overnight in warm water.

When you are ready to make the dish, drain the peanuts and beancurd. Bring a pan of water to the boil, adding star anise, Sichuan peppercorns and a pinch of salt. Add the peanuts and boil for ten minutes.

Drain and remove the spices.

In a large saucepan bring more water to the boil, plunge in the beancurd sticks and simmer for several minutes. Drain (you can reserve the water for the vegetables), cool, and pull each stick into two or three shreds before cutting into lengths of about 2cm.

Cut the celery stalks in half vertically then chop into pieces about the same length as the beancurd. Peel the carrot, cut into thin slices on the diagonal, and then halve lengthwise.

Bring some more water to the boil. Add the carrot and then the celery. Bring back to the boil, then remove with a slotted spoon. Plunge into cold water (this will preserve their bright colours). Shake excess water from all the ingredients and mix together.

Add salt and sesame oil.

There is no Chinese word for salad other than a modern transliteration, *shala*. There are numerous *liang cai*, which are cold, usually cooked, dishes. Hygiene is one of the reasons that ingredients such as beansprouts, celery and carrot are lightly blanched, but the crisp and colourful mixtures lightly seasoned with ginger, sesame oil and salt, and sometimes a splash of vinegar are also easier on the digestion and more satisfying than a mound of raw leaves. If you emulate these in your western cooking you can use one of the cold pressed oils now recognized to be full of essential fatty acids.

When I first visited the Chinese markets and tried to buy a lettuce I was surprised to find that stallholders were unwilling to sell me one, but instead tried to thrust several into my hands. It was only after studying a few restaurant menus that I realized why. Generally lettuce is served cooked in China, lightly steamed and topped with oyster sauce, stir fried with lashings of garlic, or even shredded and added to soups. Cooked green leafy vegetables can be consumed in much greater volumes than raw, so the total nutrient intake is likely to be greater than from a bowl of salad, while the seasonings create a balance of flavours. Whereas western salads are often vacuum packed or refrigerated for several days, most leaves used for Chinese cooking are fresh from the fields.

A few vegetables are eaten raw in China, including radish, both the long white one known by its Japanese name, daikon, and the large red *xin li mei* (beauty in the heart) vegetable but they are dressed with heating ingredients to help maintain a balance in the meal. Cucumber is sometimes served raw with lashings of garlic and chilli, but more often pickled or used in cooked dishes. A southern vegetable called *you mai cai* has recently become fashionable in Beijing. It looks and tastes a bit like a cos lettuce and is sometimes served raw but always with a spicy, sweet and sour dressing (see *guair wei'r*, or 'strange-flavour sauce' recipe on page 118).

Raw vegetables need spicing up because Chinese cuisine seeks a balance of *yin* and *yang*, both of flavours and of their heating and cooling energies. *Yin* and *yang*, and all opposing forces, always contain a small amount of each other. So *yin* celery is served with *yang* ginger and spring onion; crumbled dried chilli, which is hot, is added to cucumber, which is cold; *yin* ingredients such as bamboo shoots, beancurd, and mung bean noodles partner *yang* meats in stews. If the *yin/yang* balance is not found in the dish, it will be evident in the meal as a whole. Remember, anything that upsets the perfect balance between *yin* and *yang* in the body will damage Qi.

A good Chinese diet provides a natural balance. As I showed in Chapter Five, generally meats and bright coloured fruits and vegetables are *yang*, as are all the spices and seasonings, while white and light green fruits and vegetables are more likely to be *yin*, or neutral. Satisfying all five taste buds also helps achieve a balance of heating and cooling energies in the body. Pungent flavours are generally hot, bitter ones cold; sour and salty flavours are generally cool, and sweet flavours

HOT	COLD	WARM	COOL	NEUTRAL
black pepper	banana	asparagus	apple	apricot
white pepper	bitter gourd	cherry	barley	aduki beans
chilies	clam	chestnut	buckwheat	beetroot
cinnamon	crab	chicken	aubergine	carrot
dried ginger	grapefruit	chive	Job's tears (coix seed)	cashew nuts
red and green peppers	kelp	coconut juice	lettuce (very)	coconut meat
sichuan peppercorns	kiwi fruit	coriander	mango	cuttlefish
soya bean oil	mung beans	chestnut	millet	chicken egg
	mushrooms	dates	pear	fig
	octopus	garlic	sesame oil	fungus
	persimmon	lobster	beancurd	grapes
	salt	lotus root	melon	honey
	seaweed	mussels	spinach	kidney beans
	fermented soya beans	pork liver	tea	olives
	tomato	vinegar	wheat	papaya
	water chestnut	walnuts	cucumber	peas
	watercress	lamb		peanuts
	watermelon	chicken		plums
	bamboo shoot	shrimp		sunflower seeds
		onion		sesame seeds
		fresh ginger		Shitake mushrooms
		kidneys		soya bean and soya milk

9. **The heating and cooling energies of some everyday foods[14].**

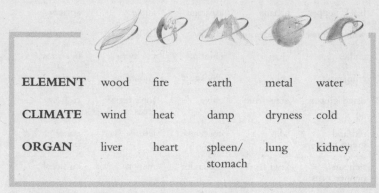

ELEMENT	wood	fire	earth	metal	water
CLIMATE	wind	heat	damp	dryness	cold
ORGAN	liver	heart	spleen/ stomach	lung	kidney

10. **The Five Climactic Conditions, the Five Elements and the Five Organs.**

tend to warm, or neutral. But because many foods combine more than one flavour the prevailing energy is not always obvious.

The problems with cold and raw foods

Watercress is a very cold vegetable. It is hard to come by in Beijing and only sold by certain traders who specialize in vegetables from the south. I would always buy a bunch if I saw it, since during my fourth pregnancy I had learned that watercress is a good source of folic acid. One day I asked the stallholder how Chinese people usually cook it. 'Only ever in soup, usually with pork,' she explained firmly. 'And you must bring the water to the boil first or it will taste bitter. Then simmer on a low heat for up to three hours.' She was obviously concerned by my look of amazement: 'Oh, and add some tangerine peel; it's a very cold vegetable you know.'

Never would watercress be eaten raw in China. Firstly, its cool properties need to be balanced by the warming orange-peel in the soup and, secondly, Chinese dietary therapy teaches that too much raw food, especially cold raw food, is damaging to the stomach because the body has to produce excess fire to digest it.

According to the Five Elements cycle there are Five Climatic Conditions: wind, heat, dampness, dryness and cold, which exist outside and inside the body. They each have a special relationship with one of the elements and the organs and, as with other manifestations of the Five Element cycle, it is important that they are kept in balance.

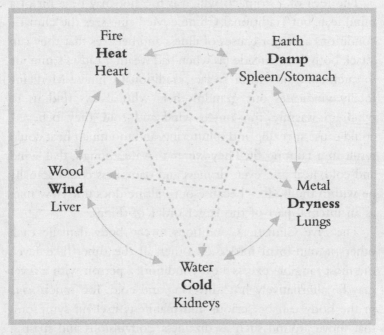

11. The Five Climactic Conditions in the Five Organs.
Solid lines show the promotion and consumption cycle, broken lines show the control cycle.

When somebody eats a lot of cold or cooling foods the body reacts by creating heat (usually described as *fire*) to consume them; if they are raw, even more heat is needed; effectively to cook them before the body can use them. If this pattern of eating becomes a habit, too much *fire* enters the stomach, which then becomes too hot and suffers from a syndrome known as *stomach fire*. If you find you cannot tolerate or do not like hot drinks, especially tea and coffee, and are often thirsty, then you are probably suffering from stomach fire. This condition can also be responsible for unaccountable hunger pangs and a host of irritating symptoms including bad breath, bleeding gums, toothache, headaches and nosebleeds.

The idea of a stomach which is too hot may be a bit of a mind leap, but Traditional Chinese Medicine sees the climatic conditions as major causes of illness and believes that they can attack both from outside (as when bad weather causes someone to catch cold) or within. In fact, Traditional Chinese Medicine totally vindicates our grandmothers who always told us to wrap up warmly. Too much wind and cold, they believed, could cause sneezing and spluttering, and too much heat could result in a fainting fit. They weren't aware, though, that wind and cold, heat and even dryness and dampness could actually be within the body – because our culture does not view man as an integral part of the larger order of things.

The Five Climatic Conditions in the body damage each other or transform into each other all the time. Take fever, the most tangible excess-heat condition: a person with a fever may be alternatively hot, shivering and cold. Too much *wind* in the body can be serious and manifests itself in symptoms that move around such as dizziness, convulsions and spasms. The climatic conditions can also attack particular organs. The stomach is especially vulnerable to *fire*, and because *fire* moves quickly and burns out it has a tendency to turn to the next climatic condition in the cycle: dampness.

The tendency of excess fire to turn to dampness explains why we need to go easy on the salad. Damp, which is associated with the earth element, and therefore the stomach, is lingering and hard to shift. So, every time we eat a salad, we create excess stomach fire, which can prevent the spleen/stomach from doing their important jobs of digesting food and distributing nutrients. Continued consumption of raw food will gradually damage the stomach *Qi* and make it unable to balance its own climate and prevent its associated element, dampness, from becoming too strong. As dampness gets out of balance, *wind*, the climatic condition that tones the spleen/stomach, attacks the body to try to remedy the situation, resulting in bloating and other uncomfortable if not embarrassing digestive upsets. Traditional Chinese medicine also sees eczema and arthritis as wind-related conditions, thus making the link between these chronic conditions and poor diet.

In China, there has never been any doubt that if a person is overweight then it is a manifestation of some deeper problem, almost universally involving dampness which has invaded their week spleen/stomach. A weak stomach also becomes vulnerable to cold, the antithesis of heat, because in the *yin/yang* scheme of things these two phenomena easily transform into the other. So, a stomach that has been under attack by *fire* for some time may eventually become a cold stomach.

Dampness in the spleen/stomach can lead to the whole body becoming too damp and dampness blocks the flow of *Qi*, leading to lack of energy or listlessness. People with a damp constitution often have a glossy tongue, sweaty palms, and a lot of what is known in Traditional Chinese Medicine as phlegm, an internal condition that can lead to high blood pressure and aching joints.

Whereas *wind* in the body tends to move upwards, *dampness* moves down. And the problems it causes can be heavy and painful, as when rheumatoid arthritis gets into the joints. Dampness can team up with heat or cold. People with a *cold, damp* constitution tend to suffer from abdominal swelling and diarrhoea, where as those with a *hot, damp* constitution have difficulty urinating and are often constipated. In extreme conditions the dampness might swing from hot to cold, and a manifestation of this effect might be irritable bowel syndrome.

In the West we usually deal with damp-related problems with a dieter's regime that almost invariably involves calorie reduction and lots of salad and raw vegetables. If the weight does shift, it may well do so at a cost. Because this regime exacerbates the problem the dampness may transform to dryness, which is why long-term dieters may suffer from poor skin, thinning hair, cracked lips, dry mouths and constipation. An undernourished body is a weak body, with damaged *Qi*. Diets can therefore leave you lacking in energy and subject to attack from within or without at any time.

Dealing with 'dampness'

For many people, learning the secrets of the Chinese diet and changing their eating habits accordingly is enough to start to shift their dampness and rebalance the body. But Chinese food therapists have particular recommendations for dampness-related obesity which do not involve complicated diet sheets or punishing regimes. Instead, they suggest eating more of certain foods that will address the particular problem. In particular, aduki beans, which are neutral in their *yin* and *yang* and their heating and cooling energies as well as being a natural diuretic, can help restore the balance in a damp body. These small red pulses are often added to *zhou* or, for a total weight loss formula, boiled with Chinese red dates to form a medicinal food that helps to strengthen the spleen/stomach. Garlic promotes the circulation of *Qi*, which can help overweight people feel more energetic. So, if you are not yet a fan of *zhou*, you can use it in your cooking. Soya beans and bean-curd are recommended for all overweight people, whether their weight problem is due to damp heat or damp cold, because they strengthen the spleen and help it to deal with the problem.

Cold, damp types need to warm their bodies to expel the excess water which may be making them feel bloated or suffer from diarrhoea. Chinese dietary therapy recommends several ingredients to help dispel cold from the stomach: dried ginger, cinnamon and dried orange-peel. Cinnamon and ginger can be ground into a powder and used in cooking or taken in a tea, and will relieve abdominal swelling. Dried ginger is more effective than fresh for this purpose. Orange-peel can be used in stews and soups or powdered for use in cooking or teas. It will also relieve other congestion or indigestion.

Other cures treat the hot, damp types, aiming to cool the body gently and naturally so that the dampness blocking the system can escape. Certain cooling foods can do this because they are known to work on the meridian lines (the channels that carry *Qi* in the body) of the spleen and/or stomach and often the heart (the source of fire) as well. These include green tea, the cucumber look-alike *ku gua* (or bitter melon, taken in soup or tea) and mung beans or beansprouts (cooked, not raw). Millet porridge also has cooling properties, which is why it is preferred to the more common rice variety by those who want

Liang cai suggestions

Chinese:	Western (or fusion):
blanched celery, 'bamboo' beancurd, carrot and boiled peanuts dressed with sesame oil and salt	cooked aduki beans (lightly stewed or marinated) mushrooms, garlic and ginger
thinly-shredded potato (blanched but crisp), strips of green chilli, sugar, salt and vinegar	boiled broccoli florets with soy sauce, pinch of sugar, sesame oil and minced garlic
blanched mung beans, toasted Sichuan peppercorns, sugar, salt, vinegar	cooked Puy lentils, roasted red pepper strips, Balsamic vinegar dressing
steamed aubergine fingers with crushed garlic, soy sauce, sesame oil and touch of vinegar	roasted or steamed sweet potato pieces with herbs, roasted cherry tomatoes, a scattering of blue cheese or beancurd dressing

to keep their external body in shape as well as their internal.

Not all cooling foods work gently to restore the balance in the body. In fact many need to be treated with caution as they worsen the situation. As much as you may crave them after a rich meal, the worst thing you can do is to bombard a hot stomach with ice cold drinks or ice-cream. These unnaturally cold foods will only cause further damage to the affected organs and the whole body.

In modern western society we quite happily put substances into our body at temperatures that our exteriors cannot tolerate. There is no place in the Chinese diet for iced drinks or frozen delicacies or for piping hot meals and beverages. There are no microwaves or hot plates to reheat food or keep it bubbling. Wok-fried or simmered dishes are placed on the table and gradually shared among the diners. By the time a small piece of food has been selected with a pair of chopsticks it is never too hot for the mouth or tongue, and so will not cause any damage to the body's equilibrium.

The formal Chinese tea-making process involves several changes of water and plenty of standing time. The resulting beverage is always served in cups without a handle so that the drinker can feel when it's ready; when it is cold enough to pick up, it is cool enough to drink. Even the famous Chinese *huang jiu*, a yellow wine made from sorghum (a type of grain), is served lightly warmed.

If you have relied on salad lunches, and possibly salad suppers, to keep your weight under control, you may be panicking at this stage. 'What *can* I eat when I want a light meal then?' I hope you have picked up some ideas throughout the book, but there is also the whole *liang cai* (cold dish) concept where vegetables are lightly blanched or steamed and mixed with a little sesame oil, salt or soy sauce, and perhaps a splash of vinegar.

Don't be dismayed to find that all those years of rabbit food and diet drinks have been doing you more harm than good. Young people, with their abundance of fire, can get away with eating more raw foods, and a salad, particularly one well dressed and with a flavour balance, will have done you more good than crisps or confectionary. Every individual has a different constitution, and individual constitutions vary according to the time of year, stage of life and even mental state. When you are fit and your *Qi* is strong you will be able to cope with extremes. But if your tolerance for physically hot or cold food is low, it is likely that your constitution is already damaged and you need to be careful.

Seek a true balance in your diet with plenty of neutral foods — fruits, nuts and seeds, pulses (especially aduki beans), beancurd as well as rice and other grain foods. Drink beverages warm or at room temperature, and lightly cook your vegetables with plenty of interesting seasonings. The tenth secret of the Chinese diet should encourage you to throw away your diet books and forget about weight loss programmes. Try, instead, to keep your body in harmony with the natural world, and do not subject it to extremes.

eleven

Use food to keep you fit

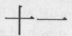

'*Yao bu bu ru shi bu*' ('Medicine will not do you as much good as food.')

ANCIENT CHINESE PROVERB

It was during a discussion with a market trader that I got my first inkling of the widespread use of home cures among the Chinese people. Every time I saw this particular woman she was very concerned to see that Sam, aged two, insisted on throwing off every article of clothing that he could work his fingers round. On Xiao Ding's instruction, I was trying to buy rock-sugar, or *bing tang* as it is known in Mandarin, but was failing miserably to explain what I wanted – both *bing* and *tang* are very common sounds in Chinese and I was having my usual problem with the tones. (I subsequently found out that I may have been inadvertently asking for 'iced soup' by mistake), and as I got more and more desperate, the crowd around me got bigger and bigger. Eventually, despairing of making myself clear through the spoken word, I tried another tack and reached into my shopping bag: 'It's to go with these pears,' I said.

'Oh,' she cried, 'you mean *bing tang*! ('Wasn't that what I said?') Your baby has a cough, hasn't he? I told you he needed to wear more clothes.' She was right on both counts. In our first year in China, I was regularly in and out of the International Medical Clinic with our third son, often to no avail. Then Xiao Ding started to suggest a few home cures, medicinal recipes that were common knowledge amongst the Chinese.

'For a cough,' she said, 'stew hard pears with rock-sugar and drink the juice. For diarrhoea, mix two eggs with water and minced ginger, steam it until it sets and top with sesame oil. For constipation, boil up sweet potato slices and drink the water. For a summer cold, drink tomato and watermelon juice and for a winter cold make a green tea with ginger and brown sugar. If in doubt, of course,' she added finally, 'eat *zhou*.'

Traditional Chinese medicine distinguishes between foods that are also medicines and herbal medicine. In China, no one has any doubt that what you eat affects the state of your health, but some foods do more than just promote well-being, they exert a specific influence on the workings of the body. Many of these foods are eaten daily and many more have been incorporated into medicinal recipes. Foods with medicinal properties, taken as part of the mixed diet nature intended, can be eaten on a regular basis without putting the body at risk.

Chinese herbalists have tested ingredients extensively on their own bodies. The most comprehensive work on actions of foods and herbs is Li Shizhen's *Ben Cao Gang Mu* (Compendium of Material Medica), which was published in 1578 and contains 2,000 entries. It was built on earlier publications, two of which, the Canon of Herbs *(Ben Cao Jing)* of Shen Nong ('the Father of Agriculture') and The Inner Canon of the Yellow Emperor, *Neijing Suwen*, date back about 2,000 years, to the Han dynasty, they were published to consolidate

the knowledge attributed to these legendary figures. The curative powers of Traditional Chinese Medicine are fascinating,
though outside the scope of this book. Many of the 'foods
that are also medicines' are packed full of health-giving properties as well as nutrients recognized by western nutritionists
– and they can be (and, in China, are) eaten every day.

A daily dose of good health

Chinese dietary therapy is all about eating foods that prevent
disease, improve health and resistance and, by toning the organs,
prolong life. Fortunately, many of the ingredients that make
Chinese food taste so delicious are also good for the body.
Ginger, spring onion and fermented black bean are believed
to expel wind and therefore help prevent common colds. Garlic
has similar properties but must be treated more carefully because
it is also classified as a medicine in Chinese thinking. Ginger
also helps digestion and disperses cold, so is used to cure many
conditions related to too much cold in the body, such as rumbling
of the intestines, diarrhoea and vomiting. Yet it is also capable
of dispersing what is known as 'superficial heat' (near the body's
surface), so is great for nausea and travel sickness. By elimi-
nating poisons it helps to make food safe to eat and was particularly valued prior to refrigeration. Chillies also promote
digestion and dispel cold. Another property of garlic is to coun-
teract toxins; if Chinese people feel that the hygiene standards
in a restaurant are poor they will chew on a few cloves.

Sichuan peppercorns, one of my favourite spices, are good
for the teeth as well as helping digestion by dispersing cold
from the stomach. The fact that Sichuan peppercorns are known
to expel roundworm is a bit of a bonus. Sesame seed, especially

the less common black variety that is often sprinkled on *zhou*, benefits the hair and lubricates the intestines. The small green mung beans clear heat from the body and are often boiled into a soup-like green porridge or made into the popular *liang pi* ('cold skin'); mung beansprouts blanched and served in cold dishes or stir-fried might be more to the western taste.

If you like to include meat in your diet, there are a number of foods that Chinese dietary therapy recommends to make its nutrients more accessible to the body and ensure that it does not stagnate in the system. White daikon radish clears blockages in the body and when combined with lamb and ginger creates a dish that nourishes the body's *yang* energy. Pork is stir-fried with lashings of coriander, which promotes digestion, or made into meat balls with minced ginger and water chestnuts, a combination that also helps eliminate congestion. In winter pork is stewed with cellophane noodles and cabbage. Cabbage stimulates the stomach and mung bean nourishes it. Hawthorn (*shanzha*) is particularly good for promoting the flow of *Qi* and is recognized by western medicine to help keep the arteries clear. It is frequently used in beef stews along with star anise, orange-peel and cinnamon, all of which help the *Qi* to circulate. Shitake mushrooms, which feature in almost all types of meat stew, as well as in soups, noodles and stir-fries, improve and strengthen the flow of *Qi,* prevent hardening of the arteries and are believed to have anti-cancer properties.

Occasionally one of my cooking school students expressed concern about the amount of oil in Chinese cooking. I was always quick to point out that in China rich fried dishes are always served alongside lighter soups and stews, but I also drew the class's attention to the many ingredients Chinese chefs use to ensure their dishes are not indigestible. *Hui xiang*, a cross

Food	Suggestions for use
Job's tears (coix seed, or *yi yi ren*)	Use in *zhou* or in minestrone style soups
rice (*mi*)	Make *zhou*. Boil, or steam and serve with *cai*; fry leftovers; use in bakes and risottos
buckwheat (*qiao mai*)	Can be boiled and served as a staple or used in bakes; or use the flour for pancakes or baking
jujube (Chinese date or *zao*)	Use in tea or *zhou*, add to soups and braised dishes; stew with dried fruit mixtures
dragon eye (*long yan*)	Delicious fresh, or the dried fruit can be removed from the stone and used as a snack, in fruit cakes or muesli or in tea
Chinese yam (*shan yao*)	Fresh can be steamed or boiled and mashed. Dried pieces can be used in soups and stewed or ground into a powder and sprinkled on soup
hawthorn (*shan zha*)	Helps the body digest meat. Use in meat stews or stewed dried fruit or add to green tea
soya beans and beancurd	Soya beans can be sprouted but should never be eaten raw, so blanch or stir-fry. For beancurd ideas see Chapter Nine
white (daikon) radish (*luo buo*)	Cut in fingers to eat raw; grate and use in soups or stir-fry with cumin and carrot
green tea (*lu cha*)	
watermelon, apple, pumpkin	

12. Foods that work on the spleen and the spleen meridian. The spleen extracts *Qi* from food, separating the pure from the impure.

Food	Suggestions for use
black sesame (*hei zhi ma*)	As a topping for *zhou*, or sprinkle on *liang cai*, or use in muesli or baking
wolfberries (*gou qi zi*; sold in the West as gouji or goji berries)	Use in tea, in chicken stock, or anywhere you might otherwise use raisins
quail's eggs (*anchun dan*)	Fry and serve on toast with roasted cherry tomatoes, or boil and serve on cocktail sticks
green tea (*lu cha*)	
oysters (*mu li* or *sheng hao*)	

13. Foods that work on the kidneys and the kidney meridian. The *Qi* from the kidneys, the body's own 'original' *Qi*, helps the heart change *Qi* into blood, which carries *Qi* round the body.

between dill and fennel, is great for the digestion. Where in the West these plants have been reduced to the status of a garnish, *hui xiang* is stuffed into the flat-breads and dumplings that are sold on every street corner in China. Another vegetable used in a similar way is Chinese chives, or *jiu cai*, which are bigger, flatter and stronger in flavour than the English equivalent: they promote the circulation of *Qi* and more specifically regulate peristalsis of the intestine.

At business meetings, get-togethers or in teahouses, walnuts are often used as a snack together with pumpkin seeds, sunflower seeds and perhaps a few sour plums, figs or marinaded quails eggs. Walnuts boost *Qi*, nourish the hair and complexion and are believed to help the brain – as they look like one. Traditional Chinese medicine worked this out long before the West

Food	Suggestions for use
lotus root (*ou*)	Usually sold dried in the West. Reconstitute, slice, blanch and dress with sesame oil, chopped spring onion and salt, or add to stews and soup
kelp (*kunbu*) (sold in the UK by its Japanese name, *kombu*)	Use in miso-style soups, add small pieces to salads or vegetable stir-fries. Helps to soften pulses when cooking
seaweed (*hai dai*)	Most Westerners find the sheets used for sushi the most palatable form
peanuts	Boil with star anise, a pinch of salt and a few Sichuan peppercorns. Add to *zhou*
pears	Use in cooking for a 'sweet and sour' flavour. Try dried as well as fresh
honey (*feng mi*)	Use in cooking or to sweeten drinks instead of sugar
lily bulb (*bai he*)	Generally only available dried in the West. Reconstitute and use in soups, *zhou*, or tea
oranges	Eat raw
garlic	Cook as lightly as possible or serve raw for full benefit

14. Foods that work on the lungs and lung meridian. The lungs take in *Qi* from the air, separating the pure from the impure. The *Qi* from the lungs then combines with the *Qi* from the spleen/stomach, and is sent to the heart.

discovered essential fatty acids and Omega-3. Sunflower seeds regulate the action of the large intestine and figs strengthen the stomach. Quail's eggs invigorate *Qi*, replenish the blood and strengthen the muscles and bones.

Foods for long life

A diet made up of the foods that nature has made available will benefit your body, especially if you use the acquired knowledge of Chinese food culture to eat them in the right combinations. I have explained how all foods tone and enter one or more organs, depending on their flavours, but some foods are also specifically recognized by Chinese dietary therapy to work on the meridians, that is, the channels which link the organs and carry the *Qi* round the body, and in doing so stimulate the flow of *Qi*. Weak or stagnant *Qi* is the precursor of disease, whereas when *Qi* flows freely, good health ensues. Because the *Qi* that circulates in the body is made up of the *Qi* that we breathe in from the air, the *Qi* we obtain from food and the *yuan*, or original *Qi* (or essence) of the kidneys that we are born with, foods that act on the lungs, spleen and kidney meridians are believed to promote long life.

The list is eclectic and there is no linking theme in terms of flavours or energies. Many of them have already cropped up before in this book for one or other of the many ways in which they promote good health. Some are easily accessible, others can only be found in specialist shops. For unfamiliar ingredients, I offer suggestions for using them both Chinese and western style (see pages 29 and 160).

Putting it all to work

Some health-giving foods are a welcome addition to any family diet, whilst others may be received with a more mixed reception. *Long yan* (dragon-eye fruit), which is similar to lychee but with smoother skin and larger stone, goes down a treat, either as a snack or in sweet or savoury dishes. *Bai he* (lily bud) is sweet and crunchy with a slightly bitter aftertaste and are always well received. Lotus root is generally a successful addition to both hot and cold dishes. The long tuber known as *shan yao*, 'mountain medicine', on the other hand, has little to recommend it in terms of flavour but can be disguised quite well in mashed potato. *Gou qi zi* (wolfberries) can be similarly hidden in carrot cake, or added to couscous along with a few raisins.

My family were quite keen on the sticky sweetened walnuts from the local market until some clever child read the packet and found out that the stickiness came from *er jiao*. Frequently used in Traditional Chinese Medicine, *er jiao*, or 'donkey-hide gelatin', is used with great effect to regulate the menstrual cycle; and although I hastily discarded them, I never heard the last of the 'donkey bottom walnuts'.

Some herbs classified as 'foods that are medicines' need to be treated with respect. I once delighted my family with Shitake mushrooms stuffed with minced chicken, wolfberries, *ren shen* ginseng and *he shao wu* (or 'multi-flowered knotweed tubers'). Tim thought they weren't bad at all, so I told him that the *he shao wu* would stop him from going grey. In the event, though, the only immediate effect of the dish was to induce a severe attack of hiccups. I also felt tight across the chest. Undeterred, I started to use the same herbs in chicken stock. Then Sam finished a bowl of noodle soup and threw it straight back up. Six trips to the bathroom later, he had recovered. *Ren shen,* ginseng, is very *yang,* and *yang,* of course, means 'upward and outward'. Speaking from experience, I advise you to use even familiar foods in moderation.

Traditional Chinese medicine

Generally, though, all the foods mentioned in this chapter can, and should, be eaten regularly to keep your body fit and well. Chinese dietary therapy can also help with specific conditions, but while you are pretty safe taking ginger tea for nausea or scrambling eggs with garlic if you have diarrhoea, I do not recommend self-diagnosis for more serious complaints. Chinese medicine is a complex subject and an illness that manifests itself in one area may be attributable to an imbalance some-where completely different. However, Chinese doctors can be found on practically every high street, and often offer a free first consultation. If you are suffering from a condition, however minor, that western medicine has not been able to cure, it may well be worth your while making a visit to one.

Traditional Chinese medicine is particularly suited to deal with chronic conditions because these are often *yin* and affect the internal workings of the body. Acute illnesses, on the other hand, are usually *yang* and shorter lived and likely to burn themselves out anyway, though when they do they may lead to a chronic condition because the body has been severely out of balance for a period of time.

Whatever your problem, a traditional Chinese doctor will look behind the obvious symptoms of an illness for a syndrome that will point to the underlying cause. You will have to describe your symptoms in great detail. Is your pain gnawing or heavy? Does it move around? Is it worse in the summer or the winter? Do you prefer hot or cold food or drinks? What time to you wake at night? Are your stools soft or hard? Is your sputum thick, thin, white or yellow? The doctor will then go on to look at the patient's tongue. Tongues are reasonably straightforward: a pale tongue represents a cold syndrome and/or *yang*, *Qi* or blood deficiency. Dark red indicates heat, and purple shows extreme heat. Taking a pulse, in the Chinese way, is a specialist job and Chinese doctors can feel nine different pulses, using three fingers at three different levels, on each wrist. Each position on the wrist corresponds to a different organ and different abnormalities can be found at different depths. 'Superficial' syndromes such as colds and minor illnesses tend to be found nearer the surface, with the more serious internal problems or damage to the *Qi* showing at a lower level.

Detailed and personal questions allow Chinese doctors to build a picture of the syndrome behind every disorder. After my daughter Honor was born I spent years feeling 'shrivelled' and, while I had had plenty of milk for the other three, I had faced a real problem feeding her. Whilst I had previously enjoyed being outdoors and especially loved to take the children swimming, I found I could no longer face the elements unless heavily wrapped up and I developed a dread of swimming pools. This was the stage when I lost my taste for hot drinks and found that alcohol stopped me from sleeping because my body seemed unable to control its temperature. Through experience I knew that if I took these minor irritations to my western-trained Beijing family practitioner, he would tell me that they were just part of getting old.

I knew that I needed a full Chinese medicine consultation, but was slightly nervous of the questions about bodily functions that I knew it would involve. Then something happened to prompt me into action: my son Sam fainted at a friend's house. It was a sweltering day in May and I was not unduly concerned; he had passed out a couple of times before and always came round fighting fit. A friend, however, was of a different opinion and before I knew it we were in the middle of a thorough investigation that involved trailing round hospitals all over town, a three-day ECG and a CAT scan.

To my great relief, but not great surprise, the western doctors found nothing serious behind Sam's fainting incident. During the investigations, however, I spent time reflecting on how many physical characteristics Sam and I shared: as child I had passed out every year or so. 'Why not take Sam along with me for a Chinese medical consultation?' I asked myself; his presence there might provide a distraction from the embarrassing questions about bowel habits that I knew to be par for the course.

In the event, they weren't even asked. Dr Li Xin was immaculately groomed with a fixed smile on his small face, and eyes that seemed to pierce right through you – and probably did.

Although he went through the motions of feeling my pulse and looking at my tongue, I think he figured me out as I entered the room. My problem, he explained, and the one that my unfortunate offspring had inherited, probably from both parents, was an excess of *yang*. Did I often suffer from nosebleeds, mouth ulcers or outbreaks of acne? How were my teeth? Did I drink wine? And did it give me a headache? What about coffee?

I wasn't convinced about his diagnosis. When I was a child I had the odd nosebleed and mouth ulcer and my share of teenage acne, but no more than most. My teeth were pretty

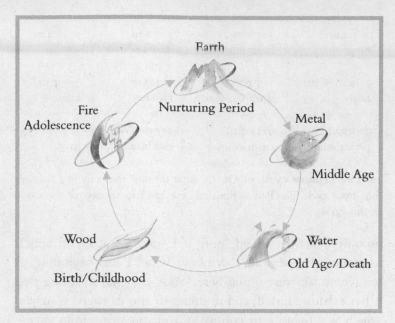

15. The Five Elements in the lifecycle.

lousy but I put that down to four pregnancies. I didn't drink any more wine than contemporaries, or most of them anyway. Yes, wine did sometimes give me a headache, as did coffee. 'But,' I asked him, to show that I had done my homework, 'I thought that if you have too much *yang* you tend to be too hot and don't feel the cold?' I had just spent most of the winter perfectly spherical from extra layers of clothing. Then I thought of something else: 'Sam never feels the cold. So how can we have the same constitution?'

Dr Li Xin patiently explained that people with excessive *yang* have too much energy; they are restless and impatient, blush easily and have a tendency to high blood pressure. Proving his point about the impatient bit, I argued with him. 'My blood pressure is very low, and so is Sam's.' Nonplussed, Li Xin asked me if I sweated a lot. 'No, hardly at all,' I announced

3–5 a.m lungs	5–7 a.m large intestine	7–9 a.m stomach	9–11 a.m spleen
11 a.m–1 p.m heart	1–3 p.m small intestine	3–5 p.m bladder	5–7 p.m kidneys
7–9 p.m pericardium	9–11 p.m san jiao	11 p.m–1 a.m gall-bladder	1–3 a.m liver

16. **The 24-hour cycle of Qi.** *Qi* flows through the body in a twenty-four-hour cycle. The Pericardium and the San Jiao are beyond the scope of this book.

proudly and then added, 'only if I wake up at night, which sometimes happens after drinking wine.' I was beginning to see where we were going here. 'Your *yang* was so strong that it has exhausted itself, and in doing so also damaged your *yin*, which was fighting to control it. You can swing from excessive *yang* to deficient *yin* at any time. When you get tired or feel low or sweat spontaneously you are displaying *yin* symptoms. When you drink wine you give your *yang* an artificial boost so you wake up sweating in the night, further damaging your *yin*,' he said.

'Because your *yin* and *yang* are damaged, your *Qi*, which is created by the balance of *yin* and *yang*, is weak which is why you cannot control your temperature or tolerate hot drinks. And you are often cold because your *Qi* is not flowing smoothly. Sam is young so he still has a plentiful supply of *Qi* to keep him warm, but as people get older their supply gets weaker, especially if they don't work to conserve it,' he explained. '*Qi* deficiency leads to weak blood, which is why your blood pressure is low rather than high and you also have problems with varicose veins and pains and numbness in your arm, do you not?' Wow.

Dr Li Xin suggested that Sam, who was in the rising *yang*

stage of his life, kept active to allow an outlet for his natural tendencies but also ate more (*yin*) sour foods to keep his rising *yang* nourished but under control. I thought about how my third son loved nothing more than to make his own home-made lemonade by squeezing fresh lemons and adding a touch of sugar. I hadn't particularly encouraged the process as it involved wielding large kitchen knives and leaving a sticky mess, but resolved to be more tolerant in future.

As for me, I took four weeks' worth of foul-tasting Chinese medicine to boost my blood and *Qi* and I underwent a course of acupuncture. I still feel the cold, but nothing like as badly as I did, and I can tolerate coffee and red wine but know to avoid too many artificial boosts to my *yang*. I incorporate plenty of foods that nourish *Qi* in my diet and have learnt to listen to my body. If it is out of sorts, however small the problem, I know it is telling me something and that I need to attempt to restore the balance, not by extreme action but by a gentle readjustment.

Read more about Chinese dietary therapy (see Further Reading on page 222) and you will find hundreds more foods with health benefits. Some of these will suit you better than others, depending on your individual constitution, your stage of life, the time of year and even time of day. In every twenty-four-hour cycle the *Qi* flows right through the body and it is at its height in the different organs at different times (see page 176).

If you always feel more out of sorts at a certain time of day, the position of the *Qi* flow in the body may be an indicator of where your weakness is. For instance, you may feel bloated in the morning, when the *Qi* is flowing through the spleen, or suffer asthma attacks in the early hours of the morning as it travels through the lung. Many people find that after a good night out they wake up at three o'clock feeling uncomfortably hot – this is exactly the time that the *Qi* passes through the liver. Alcohol is very heating, and while a youthful body can deal with its extreme effects, as we get older and our *Qi* starts to diminish we need to treat it with caution.

This ability to listen to your body is not something you can acquire overnight. If your diet to date has featured quite a limited range of foods you may find it takes time to become accustomed to, and recognize the benefits of, new tastes and textures. But if you do begin to feature some of these truly nourishing foods in your diet you will feel the difference, and your body will soon not want to return to its former undernourished state. When you get more in touch with your body you will recognise the signs that it's out of balance; these are different for every individual but could include spots, rashes, unexplained aches and pains or itching, lank hair, digestive upsets, and a host of 'allergic'-type reactions.

As I reveal the eleventh secret of the Chinese diet, that food can protect your body from disease and even treat illnesses, I am not exhorting you to rush out and stock up on quail's eggs and seaweed, nor to flush your prescribed medication down the sink. Li Shizhen's *Ben Cao Mu* (mentioned on page 164) was published in 1578, nearly 500 years ago. There are many health-giving foods available in our supermarkets today that the ancient Chinese herbalists would not have had access to. Thus, while I encourage you to seek out the foods which Chinese dietary therapy recommends, you can enjoy many other natural foods, currently promoted by today's nutritionists. If blueberries and raspberries, salmon and tuna had been available in China in the sixteenth century there is no doubt that their many health benefits would have been recognized too.

So if *er jiao* (donkey-hide gelatin) is not your thing, then look to our own food culture for foods with health benefits. In his *British Food: an Extraordinary Thousand Years of History*, Colin Spencer lists nearly one hundred wild plants that have been eaten in Britain since Roman times. Reading through the list, I could only find twenty-three that feature in every day modern-day cooking: half of those are soft fruits and nuts that until recently were used mainly for baking Christmas treats; most of the rest are herbs which are used sparingly by the initiated. Many others, including nettle, dandelion, dock and various sea vegetables still proliferate but are viewed as weeds rather than foodstuffs. Nettle helps clear toxins, dandelion improves liver function and digestion, chickweed was once used to get rid of scurvy. So next time you feel a need to go running to the chemist for a paracetamol or an antiacid tablet you might consider what's in your garden or see what the hedgerows have to offer first. There are many reliable modern guides on the medicinal properties of wild foods, and weeds.

If you only get one message from the fifteen secrets let it be this one: food is good for you. The right foods, real foods provided by nature, will help your body keep fit and free from illness.

twelve

Make an occasion of meals

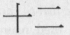

'He [the Gentleman] did not eat food that was not properly prepared nor did he eat except at the proper times. He did not eat food that had not been properly cut up, nor did he eat unless the proper sauce was available.'

CONFUCIUS, *THE ANALECTS*, C.500 BC

Chinese people enjoy food to the full, but in its right place and at the right time. Food is central to ceremonies and festivals; families and friends come together to eat at every opportunity, and no expense or effort is spared when entertaining. I have mentioned that when Chinese people eat together, the main topic of conversation is food, and there is plenty to talk about: the number of dishes, their flavour and fragrance, different ingredients and preparation methods.

Meals in China may appear complicated and elaborate compared to their western counterparts, yet attitudes to food are relaxed because everyone knows that 'appetite for food and sex is natural' (Mencius).[15] In our modern western society, on the other hand, missing meals, snacking on the run, all seem to be something to be proud of. Yet the same people who boast about not having time to eat admit (more quietly) to chocolate cravings, late-night fridge raiding, binge eating, and worse.

My grandfather used to tell me to 'breakfast like a king, lunch like a lord and sup like a pauper'. The same ideas are expressed in the Chinese saying '*zao shang chi hao, zhong wu chi bao, wanshang chi shao*' ('eat well in the morning, till you are full for lunch, and lightly in the evening'). In China most families eat their evening meal around six o'clock, sometimes even earlier. As they have generally eaten a substantial lunch, the evening meal tends to be lighter than the one we enjoy in the West, though still following the same Chinese format of several dishes with rice. Washing up is not time-consuming, a few bowls and a wok, so there is plenty of time in the evening for some kind of exercise or gentle activity.

Three meals a day in China means three meals, not two overprocessed dry snacks with a token garnish of shrivelled lettuce and something out of the microwave for supper. Often, there is little difference between the types of foods served at each meal. We have already seen the benefits of *zhou* in the morning, but breakfast is also as likely to include vegetables, protein foods and a range of flavours as in any other meal of the day.

In Beijing if you haven't time to cook you can pick up freshly made dumplings and porridge on every street corner. Beancurd sellers make a special dish called *doufu nao* out of the residue of their cottage industry. Of course, no child brought up on Coco Pops is going to change to sloppy beancurd overnight, not even if it is stewed with lily buds and wood-ear fungus. When we stayed with Guo Gui Lan in the countryside, she was sensitive to my younger children's picky eating habits and would make them piles of shredded potato and smashed cucumber to eat with their millet porridge and eggs. I lack both her single-mindedness and her dexterity with the chopper, so I'm rather less ambitious, but every day I make *zhou* for those who like it and real muesli for those who don't. On very cold days I make traditional Scottish porridge, with salt and water, not milk and sugar. And if there is any *cai* left over (sadly not that often), we eat it; cabbage and tofu, tomato and eggs, sliced mushrooms and onion are particularly popular, and I often fry up the leftover rice.

At lunch-time, the Chinese avoid eating on the run if they possibly can. Yes, they have a street food tradition, but the piles of dumplings, stuffed breads and polystyrene boxes of rice topped with *cai* sold from the street hawkers are either shared at roadside tables or taken back to work and eaten in a convivial atmosphere. While I had always been aware of the sanctity of the Chinese lunch hour, it wasn't until Liu Shifu came into our lives that I became aware of the magnitude of the issue.

Liu Shifu was a driver. Ironically, it was our move into a *hutong* (courtyard) home in the narrow streets of 'real China', a good hour's drive from my children's school, that prompted us to add him to our burgeoning household. Our new home, chosen to provide a suitable backdrop for my cooking school, was within the second ringroad that runs along the ancient foundations of the demolished walls of Beijing – and a little outside our comfort zone in China. But I knew the moment I entered the courtyard and saw the wisteria-clad walls and raised walkways that people would travel to learn in these surroundings. On the north side of the court-yard stood a spectacular room with high ceilings, ornate doors and hanging lanterns. The fact that we would have to walk outside in sub zero temperatures to reach our bedrooms seemed a minor price to pay for the privilege of such a home.

Liu Shifu joined us to take the children to school, and brought the twelfth secret of the Chinese food culture right into our *hutong* home. *Shi fu*, best translated as 'craftsman', is a polite way of addressing an adult male, but if pronounced incorrectly, as apparently was my habit, it sounds like the word for 'comfortable', so our driver was soon nicknamed 'Comfortable Liu'. It seemed an apt irony given that he was tall, thin and bony with piercing eyes and had been a martial arts champion in his youth. The name stuck and the children became fond of him, though I don't think he found his day comfortable at all since they fought incessantly as he struggled through the Beijing traffic on the journey to school.

When you employ a driver in China, he is full time. This had its advantages as Xiao Ding lived near the International School, so after he dropped off the children he would pick her up and get back just in time for the start of cooking school at 10 o'clock. The problem was, what should he do after that? Usually drivers hung out with other drivers, but we lived in Chinese *hutong* with no other foreigners around, and so no other drivers for him to pass the day with. Occasionally I would see him in the courtyard making long flowing movements but I worried that the rest of the time he must be bored out of his mind. Tim, who had found him in the first place, told me firmly, 'Give him something to do. He's much happier driving around than doing nothing.'

So I put together a list of errands and, after cooking school had finished, went to look for him. He wasn't in the kitchen or outside, nor was the car. I wandered up and down the street and was just about to go back to the courtyard to ask Xiao Ding if she could throw any light on the matter when the shopkeeper from the *xiao mai bu*, or 'little store', opposite asked me if I was looking for Liu Shifu.

I nodded assent. '*Ta chi fan qu le*,' she said, 'he's gone for lunch'. That made sense, though I was surprised that he had left it so late. 'What time did he leave?' I asked. 'Eleven thirty,' she replied, 'he always does.'

Apparently, every day he drove across to the Lido area of town, where he had formerly been based at Tim's office, to eat lunch with other members of his *dan wei*, or 'work unit'. I never tried to understand why he was entitled to this meal; my concern was more to do with the logistics. The office was a good half hours' drive from our *hutong*. 'But at lunch-time the traffic is very heavy and it might take up to an hour to get there,' Liu told me in matter of fact manner.

I discussed the whole problem with Xiao Ding, suggesting that she might knock up some fried rice or noodles for him. 'Chinese adults don't like to eat fried rice in the middle of the day; they expect a full meal – *fan* and *cai*,' she explained. 'But there are at least a dozen inexpensive good restaurants in the vicinity of this *hutong*,' I said later to Comfortable Liu. 'Can't you get lunch at one of them?' He replied that his lunch at the Lido office was free. 'But I don't mind paying,' I insisted. 'It'll be a fraction of the cost of the petrol, not to mention the wear and tear on the car.' I was getting bit hysterical.

Liu Shifu ate a couple of meals in a local restaurant but soon started to drive to his home, which was even further away than the Lido. I had paid for his meal as soon as he gave me the receipts so was still puzzled as to his motives. 'Is there a problem with the restaurant food?' I probed. No, it was fine he told me, better than at the office and much better than his wife's cooking. I realized then that I was in a classic 'China situation'. Liu Shifu could not tell me why he was not prepared to eat on his own at a restaurant because, so great was his perception of the difference between our two cultures, he knew that if I had to ask the question I would not be able to understand the answer.

The reason was that Chinese people just do not eat alone if there is any other option available. Mealtimes are not just about good food, they are about sharing good food, and company. The whole nature of the traditional multi-course Chinese meal is designed for multiple persons. My cooking school eventually employed three assistants and I noticed that it didn't matter how late they finished, they would always cook up a few dishes and eat them together. There never seemed to be any argument about what they ate, usually a medley of whatever leftovers there were in the fridge, and no one seemed to have any dislikes or even particular preferences. These everyday meals in the kitchen had the atmosphere of an informal lunch party, yet I doubted that I could carry one off with the same aplomb had I been planning it all week.

In China, the food and company generally take precedence over the table settings and the immediate environment. A small bowl and a pair of chopsticks is all that is needed for a multi-course meal. Even at formal banquets where the china is fine and chopsticks silver-plated, the array of utensils is minimalist compared to the western equivalent. This simplicity seems contradictory to the rituals and feasts of China's imperial history. But although China's emperors are famous for their elaborate banquets and ceremonies and even today formal meals can be quite a performance, these occasions are all about communication and solidarity. The overriding sentiment is that meals are about giving and sharing as much as about good food to sustain life.

More about chopsticks

Chopsticks make the Chinese dining experience and are yet another manifestation of *yin* and *yang*, as one chopstick alone has no function without the other but as a pair they make complete sense, although the two sticks have no point of contact.

The fact that chopsticks were ever introduced at all says a lot about the Chinese diet, as they are ideal for picking up roots, shoots and stems but not for hacking away at big chunks of meat. Once in use they then had a positive influence on the development of the cuisine, ensuring that all ingredients remained bite-sized and therefore easily digestible.

Using chopsticks is an art that once acquired becomes a way of life. An accomplished eater can manage to clear every grain of rice from a bowl and pick up every type of food except for liquids. Studies have shown that using chopsticks involves eighteen joints and fifty muscles: even the physical eating experience in China is holistic. Chopsticks make a meal more satisfying, and make it impossible to bolt one's food.

In the sixth century BC Confucius wrote that '*bu shi bu shi*'. The word *shi* in Chinese has several meanings, depending on how it is written or pronounced, but in this case it means 'time' and 'food'. Confucius meant here that 'If the time is not appropriate you should not eat.' Of course, China does have its street and snack foods, but these generally offer healthy and freshly prepared savoury treats which are never regarded as a preferable alternative or even an adequate substitute for a real meal.

The harmony of Chinese cuisine is a reflexion of traditional Chinese culture. People may have different opinions, interests or attitudes but they come together at regular intervals and share the same food in a warm and positive atmosphere. The foods enjoyed at Chinese festivals symbolize unity. I have already described how families mark the advent of the New Year by wrapping *jiaozi* dumplings and how they enjoy the round *yuan xiao*, stuffed rice flour balls, on the first full moon of the year. The other major festivals of the year are the Dragon Boat Festival on the fifth day of the fifth lunar month and the Mid-Autumn Moon Festival. All across China on these dates people enjoy the same foods. The Dragon Boat Festival is celebrated with *zongzi*, reed leaves stuffed with glutinous rice with a mixture of fillings that tend to be sweet in the north (Chinese dates or red bean paste) and savoury in the south (eggs and pork). In mid-autumn people enjoy 'moon' cakes filled with nuts, lotus seeds, bean paste and other delicacies, to celebrate the end of the harvest, the brightness of the moon at that time and the coming together of *yin* and *yang*. For in China, the sun personifies *yang*, the source of light and heat, while the moon is *yin* darkness and moisture; at the Moon Festival the two come together as summer heat gives way to autumn coolness.

The Chinese adherence to the lunar calendar, which fixes dates according to natural phenomenon, perpetuates people's connection with the natural world. There is a pattern to life in China, and this transmits itself into daily routine, even to something as simple as eating regular meals.

Making it work for you

Like the other changes I have recommended for your diet, the incorporation of three real meals into your daily routine is not something you need to accomplish overnight, or stick to rigidly. Nor is it likely that you will be able to make an occasion of every one. But with your new awareness of Chinese food culture you may find you are already moving towards this pattern. And as you grow in confidence you will be able to invite others to share it with you.

thirteen

Drink green and herbal teas

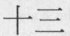

'[Green tea] opens up the avenues of the body, promotes digestion, removes flatulence and regulates body temperature.'

LI SHIZHEN (1518–93)

On one of my early visits to China I had the good fortune to be taken on a visit to a factory that made rubber car parts on the outskirts of Beijing. Heralded as a 'foreign expert' I had to sit through a two-hour meeting in a drafty room without the foggiest notion of what was going on. The only diversion, apart from a glossy photo of a sandy beach with an emerald-green sea, was a chipped, lidded mug full of a pale yellow liquid, with a few floating leaves that was topped up as quickly as I could down it. Such was my introduction to Chinese tea, and I was immediately impressed with its powers. Despite being badly jet lagged and three months pregnant, I managed to see the meeting through to its conclusion without falling asleep.

Chinese tea is green tea. It originates from the same plant as the black tea (*Camellia sinensis*) that is generally enjoyed in the West as a milky brew, but its leaves undergo less processing. Legend has it that Chinese tea (*cha*) was discovered by Shen Nong, 'the Father of Agriculture', who spent his life tasting wild plants to see their effect on the human body. One day, having eaten some poisonous plants, he picked some tea-leaves, brewed them in a pottery tripod and drank the liquid. The toxins disappeared from his body.

Originally viewed as a medicine, tea gradually became popular as a drink among Chinese scholars who found that it cleared the mind and gave them inspiration. Unlike Chinese food culture, which has its origins in the habits of ordinary people, tea drinking first found favour among the educated, the powerful and even the wealthy. In an environment at risk from dissension, corruption and extravagance tea represented tenacity, purity and simplicity, the *yin* to counterbalance the *yang*. There is no doubt that it has role to play in modern society.

In the famous *Classic of Tea*, written by Lu Yu in the Tang Dynasty (eighth century), tea is claimed to be an important elixir of immortality. Lu Yu's book contains ten chapters and covers everything from the origin of tea and where best to grow it, to how to make it and appreciate it. But more than this, it makes tea-drinking into an art form, creating the concept of the tea ceremony and a tea culture. Most importantly of all, it attributes a moral aspect to the art of tea-drinking, using it as a manifestation of the Taoist belief that man is an integral part of nature.

During the Tang dynasty the ten main benefits of Chinese tea were thus summarized:

1. Improves health and relieves headaches and fatigue
2. Helps dispel the effects of alcohol
3. Allays hunger

4. Keeps the body cool in summer
5. Prevents drowsiness
6. Can purify the mind and dispel worries
7. Helps digest greasy food
8. Eliminates toxins from the body
9. Promotes long life
10. Aids self-knowledge.

If I haven't convinced you to put the kettle on perhaps the findings of modern scientists will. Two thousand years ago the Chinese people found out what modern research is just beginning to unveil: our bodies need protection from the ravages of nature, and one of the best forms of protection is provided by nature itself. It is now known that a by-product of the metabolic process, free radicals or 'highly reactive molecules', are involved in the progression of many modern killers, including heart disease and cancer, and are responsible for much of the ageing process. Plants contain substances called anti-oxidants, which allow them to mop up the excess free radicals that are produced when they absorb energy from the sunlight. Animals don't produce anti-oxidants in the same way, so they need to eat plants – which is why the Chinese soon worked out that 'vegetables are the dishes'. But it is simply not possible to consume sufficient volumes of plant material to obtain all the anti-oxidants we need – and in any case, some of the best sources of anti-oxidants are not particularly palatable.

Green tea is made from the young buds of the leafy bush, which are carefully picked and dried immediately by a light steaming or firing process. Natural enzymes present in the freshly plucked leaves cause them to auto-oxidize, but this process is checked by the gentle heat so that the anti-oxidants in the leaves are preserved. In black tea, on the other hand, the auto-oxidation process goes unchecked, producing a darker colour and stronger flavour but also destroying some of the anti-oxidants.

Millions of Chinese people start the day by putting a pinch of dried tea-leaves in an old jam jar and adding hot water. They keep it with them, confident in the knowledge that, wherever they go, they only have to ask and someone will dig out a flask and top it up with boiling water.

I had first enjoyed Chinese tea with my young teacher, Hong Yun. When the confines of her small apartment became too restricting we would take our books to a small teahouse overlooking the lake in Tuan Jie Hu (Union Lake) park. Like all true Chinese tea-houses, our retreat did not serve food, apart from the odd dish of melon seeds, dried figs or boiled peanuts; the tea experience needs no complement.

Hong Yun was young and trendy and she was a fan of plain green tea, *lu cha*. Older Chinese people often favour the flower or jasmine tea called *hua cha*, which has flowers added to the leaf before drying. It was many years before I ceased to be daunted by the amazing array of varieties and grades of tea or to appreciate the differences. I was fortunate in my time in Beijing in that tea is probably the most regularly given gift by Chinese visitors, and as we held an open house our shelves were stocked with some of the top grade teas in China.

China's finest green tea is from the hills beside the West Lake in the eastern city of Hangzhou. I visited this scenic area when my children were aged ten, eight, four and eighteen months. As our bus wound its way up the hazardous road I occasionally relaxed enough to marvel at the endless terraces with their neatly pruned bushes.

During the evening entertainment of karaoke and ballroom

dancing that is an essential part of such expeditions, I nursed my tall glass of fine green leaves, noticing how they stood upright on the bottom. The distinctive characteristic of Hangzhou's *Long Jing* (Dragon's Well) tea is that the leaves are flat, rather than rolled, which leads to this unusual presentation of the drink itself.

It is unlikely that you will be able to adopt the Chinese tea habit overnight. I didn't really take more than the occasional cup until I started to use up my supplies by serving green tea in my cooking school. A few diehards would demand coffee instead, but I made many a convert, myself included.

Unlike tea and coffee, which provide a quick fix often followed by a let down, green tea is refreshing, thirst quenching and gently stimulating. As well as being worthy of the most special occasion, and even its own ceremony, Chinese tea can be an anytime drink. I too adopted the jam-jar habit until the day that I turned up with it at a parent–teacher conference and the children started a list of 'embarrassing things that my mother has done'. The jam-jar, it appeared, was even worse than giving lectures on Chinese vegetables to fellow parents or putting Shitake mushrooms in their lunch-boxes.

There are hundreds of varieties of green tea, but it is not the only health-giving infusion in China. A Chinese tea-shop is a true Aladdin's cave. Colourful flower teas promise subtle and delicate flavours: rose buds are believed to sooth menstruation and cure stomach pains; chrysanthemum (to be used in moderation) cools the body. Grain teas are an economical option: barley helps digestion and recovery from heat exhaustion; corn promotes urination.

Nutritional supplements are big business in the twenty-first century. With their extensive knowledge of the curative powers of natural ingredients, Chinese herbalists had the same idea centuries ago, but instead of packaging therapeutic ingredients in silica capsules they served them in teas. I have already discussed how nutrients in liquid form are particularly effective, and a cup of herbal tea also serves as a tasty drink. Understanding that nature never intended micronutrients to work in isolation, and that different types of people have different tastes and needs, the Chinese herbalists, over the years, devised a number of combinations based on the Chinese concept of eight treasures, or *ba bao*. The various flavours and properties of the 'eight treasures' in *ba bao cha* (eight treasures tea) are harmonized by a few lumps of rock-sugar. (Unlike refined white sugar rock-sugar is believed to have many benefits to health and not contribute to weight gain.) If you are fortunate to have access to a good oriental supermarket or Chinese medicine store you can try *ba bao cha* for yourself, and possibly get advice about which variety is most appropriate for your constitution.

Although the ingredients of eight-treasure tea vary, the key ones, which are pretty universal, are all now recognized in the West to have benefits for health. You will also recognize them from the list of foods to prolong life mentioned in Chapter Eleven, as they are important foods in Chinese dietary therapy. Added to green tea, they enhance its health benefits with flavour. Hawthorn, *shan zha,* provides additional anti-oxidants that have anti-viral, anti-bacterial and anti fungal properties. Wolfberries (*gou qi zi*) have been heavily marketed in health food shops in recent years, as they are one of the richest sources of vitamin A and iron. The Chinese date or jujube (*da zao*) is an unassuming fruit that grows abundantly in the hills around Beijing but is bursting with micro-nutrients, including Vitamin C and several B-vitamins as well as a host of anti-oxidants to fight those free radicals. Dragon fruit (*long yan*) is also packed full of vitamins, including B1, B2, C, and amino acids.[16] Then there are lotus seeds, lily buds, dried apricots, or stronger herbal ingredients such as ginseng.

Chinese herbalists did not isolate vitamins, let alone fatty acids and anti-oxidants, but they knew a lot about the curative powers of natural ingredients, much of which the West has yet fully to understand. Hundreds of folk stories exist promulgating the benefits of Chinese herbal ingredients. There is the story of the stepmother who tried to kill her stepchild by feeding him under-cooked rice, but because the child feasted on hawthorn berries (*shan zha*) from the fields every day, he did not even suffer from indigestion. Then there is the tale of the defeated army cut off and stranded on the mountain, surrounded by their conquerors. It was assumed that they would starve to death, but instead they survived by eating 'mountain medicine' (*shan yao*) and a year later reappeared and scored a decisive victory. The details may be blurred or exaggerated, but the messages are clear.

And like the other secrets of the Chinese diet, the tea habit is one that you can adapt to your own tastes and lifestyle. Many western herbal teas are bursting with health benefits, some make use of Chinese therapeutic ingredients: ginger and fennel help digestion, as does liquorice, which is also an energy tonic. Cinnamon is warming, peppermint is cooling. Then there are European plants: nettle cleanses the liver and is a mild laxative, camomile is a sedative, and verveine a nervous tonic. All these options, and green tea, are now available from most supermarkets and more and more food and beverage outlets are providing them too. Look out for loose teas if you can find them since the teabag varieties are inferior to the fresh – with green tea in particular, they are usually made from the 'dust' which remains after the whole leaves have been boxed. But any green tea is better than no green tea.

Think of these drinks as an addition to your usual routine. Have them on hand to quench your thirst or fill an idle moment. As your body begins to feel the benefits you may find that the caffeine-loaded stimulants you have relied on until now begin to lose their appeal.

fourteen
Take restorative exercise

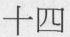

'In the past people practised the Tao, the Way of Life
. . . combining stretching, massaging and breathing to
promote energy flow. . . thus it is not surprising that
they lived over one hundred years.'

FROM *NEIJING SUWEN*, THE INNER CANON
OF THE YELLOW EMPEROR OR HUANG DI;
CIRCA SECOND CENTURY AD

My daughter Honi, when aged three, once asked me why
there were so many old people living in China. This foxed
me for a moment, until I realized that what she was really
talking about was not an issue of demographics but of lifestyle.
In Beijing, old people almost exclusively live in their com-
munity, and they are very evident. Whether they are sitting
in the streets playing mahjong, or congregating with others
in the park, bringing caged birds whose song provides a background for their morning get–together, they make full use of
their retirement, exercising body and mind gently. They

frequently carry two round metal balls, which they manipulate gently with their hands so that they keep the joints supple and the *Qi* flowing.

As well as the post-prandial stroll which is a way of life in the summer months, some people do better and attend ball-room dancing classes. I noticed that even the fast modern-ization of Beijing did not deter people from getting out and about. Ballroom dancing classes often took place under the flyovers of the third ring road, and it was not unusual to see people running backwards (to stimulate the brain) along the hard shoulder of the airport motorway.

Daily exercise routines focus on suppleness, control and coordination. On summer evenings families venture out together to fly colorful paper kites, which can be bought inexpensively all over the city. After dark these incorporate small lights. I particularly remember one balmy evening when, looking up into the sky and seeing a myriad of red dots shining in the dark sky, I ventured out to find the source. The tran-quillity of the scene, among the debris of a nearby development area, was extraordinary.

In order to understand the Chinese attitude to exercise we need to revisit the concept of *Qi*, or life-force, and recall the fact that our supply diminishes as we get older. Why on earth then would we want to punish our bodies with rigorous exercise routines that reduce our supply of *Qi?* 'To burn up more calories,' you will cry in response – until you remember that the way to a fit and slim body is not through counting calories, but through balancing our diets Chinese style so that we nourish all our organs.

Before you skip this chapter with a sigh of relief that you don't have to add a daily workout to the porridge and beancurd regime, recall that a healthy lifestyle is all about moderation.

Regular gentle exercise is a good thing. The rhythm of everyday Chinese life starts with early morning activities in Beijing's parks and open spaces, or cycling to work, which is a necessity for many. The Chinese way of exercise is generally gentle and sustaining. Young people take part in competitive sports and train intensively. Teenagers play table tennis and basketball, but as people get older they do so with dignity. People of all ages play badminton in the street. As well as the evening outings there are early-morning Tai Chi groups in every park, dancing lessons involving colourful flags and early-morning stretching exercises. None of these activities involves any special clothing or equipment.

Qi gong

Chinese exercise routines keep both body and mind in shape. All the Chinese, and other Asian forms of martial arts, are based on an ancient practice called *Qi gong*. Like many other Chinese terms, *Qi gong* defies exact translation. You should, however, already be comfortable with the concept of *Qi*, and *gong* translates reasonably as 'exercises', 'work', or 'skill', so *Qi gong* means to work the life-force. *Qi gong* teaches ways to move and breathe in order to help the *Qi* work in the body and strengthen all its organs.

Qi gong is one of the many legacies of Laozi, (the father of Taoism), in whose teachings the ideas of balance and harmony are so clearly expressed. The perfect man, in Taoist writings, achieves *yin/yang* harmony: 'In repose he shares the passivity of the *yin*, in action the energy of the *yang*.'[17]

Modern exercise routines are generally *yang*: they may tone our outer shape and speed up our metabolism, but because *yang* is everything that is heating and outwards moving, when we finish a workout we are likely to be red-faced and sweaty. As we work to tone our stomachs, thighs and buttocks, we are ignoring the more *yin* aspects of our bodies: the organs, the blood and the bodily fluids (the Chinese term for all internal liquids including saliva, gastric juices, phlegm, tears, mucus and sweat). And as we know an excess of *yang* will damage *yin*.

When Dr Li Xin diagnosed my *Qi* deficiency I questioned him: 'It can't be that bad. I'm pretty fit. I work out in the gym for an hour three to four times a week and I can run for an hour. I've done years of aerobics classes and always manage to keep going, no matter how tough the workout.' Dr Li Xin smiled. 'That's your *yang* pushing you, not your *Qi*.'

Qi gong works both the *yang*, through movement, and the *yin*, through breathing. Every movement is balanced with *yin* and *yang* aspects. Control of the breathing, or respiration, is crucial to successful practice. Exhalation, or expiration, is *yang*, while inhalation, or inspiration, is *yin*. The common uses of the technical terms 'expiration' and 'inspiration' say it all. As we go through life we put out more than we take in, until the day when we give out our last breath. If we were to concentrate, instead, on the inspiration, our minds would be clearer, our bodies healthier and our lives longer.

Qi gong does just that – the movement is the method – but the ultimate is a state of inactivity or meditation where the *Qi* can flow freely through the meridians and circulate around the organs. The power of *Qi* is so strong that experienced practitioners can harness their own *Qi* to heal others. Like other branches of traditional Chinese healing, *Qi gong* needs to be carried out by someone who knows what he is doing; even self-practice is better learnt from a master. However, there are some simple routines you can try for yourself and which may fill that space that you previously reserved for the gym, and leave you time to spare. And unlike the gym, the practice of *Qi gong* doesn't involve any special clothes, mats or equipment, just a comfortable outfit and enough space to turn round.

By stimulating your *Qi* flow you are helping your body to exercise itself. If the *Qi* is flowing freely the body will keep fit. The best time to practise *Qi gong* is between five and seven in the morning, when the *Qi* is flowing through the lungs, but before breakfast is good enough – or any time you have peace and quiet, so long as it is not straight after a meal, when the body is busy digesting.

I studied *Qi gong* at the Beijing University of Traditional Chinese Medicine. Our mentor, Professor Song, positively exuded good health as he performed movements with the strength and control of a young athlete even though he must have been at least sixty-five. I have clear memories of sunny spring mornings in the university gardens with its pagodas and wisteria-clad walkways. But at the time I was surprised to discover that more than half the class took place within the classroom where we learnt about the relationship between the Five Organs and the Five Flavours and how to view the human body in terms of the Five Elements. It was only when this concept was in our grasp that we could start to understand how *Qi* moves around the body via meridians and how, by encouraging this *Qi* to flow freely, we could enhance our overall health.

There are certain points on the body where the *Qi* flows nearer to the surface. The movement of *Qi* can be improved by stimulating these points through acupuncture, acupressure and massage, all of which are branches of Traditional Chinese Medicine. Western medics are at last taking these alternative therapies more seriously, but a little known secret is that it is

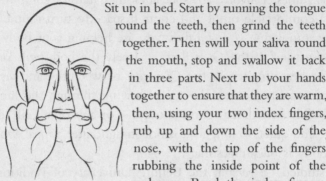

Sit up in bed. Start by running the tongue round the teeth, then grind the teeth together. Then swill your saliva round the mouth, stop and swallow it back in three parts. Next rub your hands together to ensure that they are warm, then, using your two index fingers, rub up and down the side of the nose, with the tip of the fingers rubbing the inside point of the eyebrows. Bend the index fingers, close your eyes and, using the backs of the fingers, rub the lids across and back. Open your eyes and move the eyeballs in the socket both clockwise and anti-clockwise.[18]

Traditional Chinese medicine teaches that the health of the whole body is reflected in the ear. If this sounds a little extreme, feel inside your ears next time you have a hangover or are feeling under the weather. You will probably find a small, hot pimple or a tender spot. So, in pursuit of better health, take hold of one ear with each hand, rub them both all over and pull at the lobes.

Next run your fingers from your forehead back across your head, right down to the neck. Cover your face with your palms and rub down and round. Still in bed, turn your head from left to right to loosen the neck. Massage the left shoulder blade with the right hand and the right shoulder blade with the left. Punch the air in front of you with alternate fists. Then rub your kidneys (lower back). Lie down and rub the stomach (clockwise if you tend to be constipated and anti-clockwise if you are more likely to suffer from diarrhoea – or alternate if you have no problems in that area).

Now it is time to get out of bed. Stand with your feet at shoulder width, bend your knees slightly and rotate the hips in a circular motion. Sit back on the bed, if you wish, and rub the knees. Then massage each foot, starting by pulling the toes, press hard into the ball, and work right back to the heel and ankle. The foot is another mirror of the whole body, and if you find you have tenderness in any particular area you would do well to try a foot massage – a qualified reflexology practitioner may be able to tell you if the discomfort is a manifestation of a more serious problem elsewhere in the body.

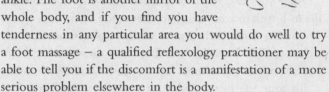

This simple full body massage routine will take between ten and twenty minutes, depending on how many repetitions you do, and will set you up for the day.

18. *Wu Xing Zhang* – Five Elements Palm tech-

Wu Xing Zhang

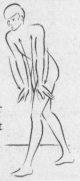

Following the Five-Elements cycle, start by toning the liver, the *wood* element. This exercise should be practised more in the spring. Stand facing east with your legs at shoulder width apart and your palms touching in front of your chest. Breathe in as you step back on to your right leg, straightening your left. Twist your body to face left and move your arms down towards the knee, palms down, then turn the palms in towards the body and make a scooping motion as you bring the hands up until they reach shoulder height. Start to breathe out, making the healing sound 'shuuuuuuuuu', and push the palms out, then down again, transferring your weight onto the front knee, as the arms lower back towards it. When the hands reach the knee, breathe in again, scoop the arms up, straighten the front knee and bend the back. Repeat the movement complete with healing sound, at least twice.

After you have finished your left-facing movements, use the in-breath to accompany another scooping motion where you swing your body round to the right, straighten the right leg while bending the left one and carry out the exercise above the right knee, for the same number of times.

To tone the heart, shift your position so that you face south. Let the arms hang down, elbows rounded, palms facing upwards, and fingers lightly touching. With the feet slightly more than shoulder width apart, bend both knees, lift the hands up to shoulder height and breathe in. Straighten the left leg and lean back on to the right, push the arms out to the left at shoulder level with the palms facing outwards. Rock forward on to the left knee and then take your weight over both knees in a squatting position as you bring the hands round to the right in circular motion, breathing out with the sound 'hurrrrrrr'.

When your hands reach the far right, breathe in as you bring them down and turn the palms upwards as you straighten the right leg and rock back onto the left. You can then repeat the movement in the other direction and continue to alternate directions for as many repetitions as you like, but at least three on each side.

To tone the spleen, stay facing south. Put the feet together and let your fingertips touch, palms facing upwards. Breathe in and lift the right arm up at the same time as you lift and bend the right knee. As the hand reaches your chest, move the arm out to the side as you turn the palm over to face the ground. You will then be balancing on the left leg with the right arm outstretched. As you bring the arm down to the centre, and the leg to the ground, breathe out with a 'hoooooooo' sound. Repeat with the left arm and left leg; then alternate sides at least twice more.

In order to tone the lungs, step the right leg round so that you are facing west. Breathe in, take your weight back on to the right leg, bending the right knee while lifting your arms up to chest height and pulling the right arm back and shooting the left forwards, just as if pulling a bow and arrow. Then 'release the bow': pull the left arm into your chest and shoot the right arm forwards, straightening the back (right) knee and bending the front (left). Breathe out with a 'suuur' noise during this movement. Pull back and breathe in. Repeat the whole movement at least twice, then swing to the right and carry out the same movement in reverse.

Finally, to tone the kidneys, step round so that you are facing north. Stand with the legs comfortably apart, breathe in and lower to a squatting position, taking the weight back on to the right leg, bending the right knee and straightening the left. Keep your hands low, palms to the floor. Then breathe out and, making the sound 'chway', rock forward on to the left leg. Lift the arms slightly up and pull the palms up, then turn them over to face the ground in a lifting and falling movement and, settling into a squat, move the hands in a circular motion from left to right until the weight is over the right leg. Lean back onto the left leg, pull the arms up and round and breathe in then repeat the movement at least twice.

According to the Five-Elements theory, each movement corresponds to a season and should be performed more often at the appropriate time. So, the liver needs more toning in spring, the heart in summer, the spleen in late summer, the lungs in autumn and the kidneys in winter. But the movements are best carried out as a sequence, so just increase the repetitions for the organ that needs more toning at any particular time. Once you are experienced, you will find that the movements flow naturally from one to the other in accordance with the Five-Elements cycle.

19. Standing Meditation

Face south with the feet shoulder width apart, relaxing the knees and hips. Tuck your tailbone in, relax the pelvis, straighten the back but allow the shoulders to droop slightly. Bend the elbows, then allow them to droop; move the arms slightly away from the body so that the armpits are open and hollow; relax the wrists. Lift the head until you can imagine it hanging from a thread above the body; tuck in the chin. Close the eyes lightly, and touch the lips and teeth together. Finally lift up the tip of the tongue so that it touches the upper palate. This small movement forms a bridge so that *Qi* can circulate around the meridians that run vertically through the body.

In this position you should be able to concentrate on your breathing, especially when you inhale (remember the technical term, inspiration) and on the *dantian*, a point about three fingers' width below the navel. Traditional Chinese medicine teaches that this is the starting point of the circulation of *Qi* and the place where *Qi* is stored.

When standing you should let your thoughts slip away: acknowledge them and let them pass by, all the time bringing your attention back to the flow of *Qi*. After a time your mouth may fill with saliva, you may feel warm or even start to sweat – these are all signs that the *Qi* is flowing. After your standing meditation, which you can practise for between two and fifteen minutes, rub your hands together, then shake lightly to get rid of any tensions.

perfectly possible to stimulate many of these points oneself. In fact many Chinese people do so every day, starting before they even get out of bed, although if you live with a partner you may prefer to find a private place since not all the exercises can be done in silence!

The following self-massage routine can be performed on its own but ideally should be followed by the *Wu Xing Zhang* (Five Elements Palm Technique), which tones the Five Organs, and a short period of standing meditation. Each action should be performed at least thirty-six times, though you can do as many as a hundred if you have time.

The *Wu Xing Zhang* that follows is a series of linked movements with 'healing sounds' that tone the Five Organs, by purifying their *Qi* and dispelling toxins so that your whole body is fit and ready to go. Traditional Chinese medicine has focused on the sounds that we make naturally to stimulate the body's innate healing capacities. If you think this sounds a bit far-fetched, remember that human beings have always made noises when experiencing emotions, and I will show in the next chapter how the emotions are linked to the organs. Children scream when they are angry or excited; the screaming sound is linked to the liver. We all know that talking can release tension, and this is particularly true where the energy of the spleen is disrupted, since the spleen is associated with worry and stress. If we can rebalance our organs we can digest food better and shift excess weight. It must be worth a try.

Conclude the *Wu Xing Zhang* with a period of standing or meditation. During meditation the mind is emptied of all thought and the body stops responding to external stimuli, enabling it to restore its own balance. Successful practice enhances the metabolism and boosts the immune system. In

China, parks are full of men and women moving gracefully in a trance-like state, oblivious to the buzz of city life but totally aware of their place in the natural order of things.

The passivity of yin *and the energy of* yang

Meditation does not come naturally to me. I have never been very good at switching off. The truth is that, like many people in the West, I find the thought of a day with nothing to do rather threatening. If I ever look ahead and see an empty schedule, I feel a bit panicky and my first reaction is to rush to the phone or send a few e-mails. I suspect that at heart I am really a couch potato and that if I let myself experience a period of inactivity I might find that I like it.

The body's state of activity is *yang* and inactivity is *yin*. When I came to understand that *yin* and *yang* always contain at least small amounts of each I recognized that I am a potentially lazy person inside an obsessively busy one, and that fear of this other side of my nature had made me push myself unnecessarily. Had I let my body rest more, especially after I had asked a lot from it, I would be a fitter person. In China, women stay inside for a whole month after giving birth (a process that demands a tremendous amount of one's *Qi*). During this time they have the support of the extended family and lots of nourishing soup. Traditionally, new mothers did not even change their clothes and great care was taken to maintain their body at an ambient temperature. Breastfeeding is still seen as a full-time occupation, not something that you do in your lunch break, as I had done.

It is never too late to start on a programme of restorative exercise and meditation. By practising *Qi gong* you will begin to build a healthier relationship between yourself and your body, between yourself and nature and ultimately between yourself and the world. Regular and sustained practice will help build your inner strength; if you are not in control of your eating, it will help by strengthening your willpower. But also, as you balance the *yin* and *yang* and the Five Elements in your body and in your organs, you will find that you naturally seek out truly nourishing foods. The *Qi gong* routines I have outlined here are just an introduction to this age-old practice. But the best way is to join a class. *Qi gong* is not usually taught in the West, but the related martial art form, Tai Chi, is increasingly popular. More about physical balance than inner harmony, it is nevertheless a way in to restorative exercise.

The calories in versus calories out approach to diet and exercise puts tremendous strain on mind and body alike. Your exercise routines, like your diet, should be sustaining and nourishing, enhancing your *Qi*, not exhausting it. All you need to do this is to improve the way you breathe. A brisk walk in the country or a session on the dance floor can make you feel great, not because you have burnt up 200 calories but because you have filled your body with the *Qi* from the air. With practice you will be able to achieve the same sensation through mediation. When the lungs sort the pure from the impure and the *Qi* joins with that we ingest from the earth via our food and that of our own essence, the basic life processes are vitalized. As we breathe out, exhaling substances that will nourish the plants we eat, we take our place in the natural order of things and renew our relationship with the rhythm of the universe.

If your chosen form of exercise makes you feel good then it is likely to be doing you good. Be aware that your body is more than just tissue and muscle. The right type of exercise, like the right diet, will help keep you fit inside and out. If you are totally exhausted after visiting the gym, or running five miles, then your session may have done more harm than good to consider alternatives. A survey carried out by Cancer Research showed that women who do their own housework are 30 per cent less likely to suffer from cancer than those who don't.[19] The results of the survey showed that moderate forms of physical activity may be more beneficial to health than less-frequent but more intense recreational activity (e.g. going to the gym). According to the Five Elements concept, cleaning and polishing tones the metal element, keeping us fit into old age. Or what about digging the garden and sowing some fresh organic vegetables? You would not only tone your wood element, but you would contribute towards the scheme of things and enhance your own diet at the same time. Another Chinese proverb says '*zhi you yi hao*' ('everyone has his or her own preferences').

fifteen

Avoid extremes in all areas of your life

十五

> '*Gong tai man ze zhe; yue tai man ze que.*' ('When a bow is pulled too far it will break; when the moon is at its fullest, it will wane.')

OLD CHINESE PROVERB

The Chinese saying '*suan, la, tian, ku*' ('sour, spicy, sweet and bitter') doesn't refer only to the flavours of Chinese food but is used to describe the emotions in a truly fulfilling life.

The connection between illness and emotional state is so often overlooked in the West. We might admit to being run down or stressed out, but these states are almost seen as something to be proud of. If we were to admit that illness might result from an imbalance in our lifestyle, then we would have to acknowledge we are responsible for doing something about it.

There are five indigenous pathogens or emotions, as they are called in Traditional Chinese Medicine, linked to the Five Elements and Organs, and with the same creation and control cycle. Like the flavours, the right amount of emotion exerts a positive effect on an organ; too much can cause damage.

ELEMENT	wood	fire	earth	metal	water
ORGAN	liver	heart	spleen/stomach	lungs	kidney
EMOTION	anger	joy	worry/thought	grief	fear

20. **The relationship between the Five Elements, the Five Organs and the Five Emotions.**

According to Chinese thought, too much anger, associated with the liver, makes the Qi rush upwards, too much joy (heart) upsets its smooth circulation. Too much worry or thought (spleen) can make the Qi stagnate, excessive grief (lung) can consume it and extreme fear (kidneys) will force Qi downwards.

Living in China has made me acutely aware of the different pressures of modern and traditional lifestyles. In underdeveloped areas, people are not so insulated from negative emotions. People in many regions of China live in constant dread of natural or man-made disaster. Floods are commonplace and the country has a history of tragic earthquakes; the newspapers report a fatal accident in mines at least once a month. I have seen factories in China where the conditions make the Victorian age look state of the art. There was a family living in a hut with no sanitation or electricity less than a mile from our home. They had moved up to Beijing to work the land there because, back home in Hebei about 300 miles south, there wasn't enough to eat. The Chinese are no strangers to the concept of *chi ku* (or eating bitterness), and believe that a period of hardship has its place in the scheme of things.

Children seem to be able to cope with extremes of emotion; they are in their wood stage of life, with plenty of rising *yang*. As we get older our bodies are not so forgiving. Too much anger, especially when bottled up, might manifest itself in liver malfunction, leading to headaches and migraines; excess worry can damage the spleen/stomach and leads to abdominal bloating and problems with the digestion.

In the West, grief and fear are often experienced only vicariously through TV and films, only to be all the more overwhelming when they do strike home. My solution over the years has been to enrol all my children in aggressive, competitive sports in the hope that the pre-game tension, adrenalin flow and after-match emotion might add balance to their relatively charmed existence. As the older boys entered their teenage years, I was unsure that a weekly game of ice hockey was enough. Beijing is a teenager's dream: beer is cheap, taxis are cheap, and there are no licensing laws or age restriction on nightclub entry.

When our eldest son, Max, opted at the age of thirteen to spend a year at a local Chinese school called the Number Fifty-five Middle School, his ex-pat teenage life was put into perspective. As Christian neared the same age, he made it perfectly clear that, thanks to Max's reviews of the establishment, he would not be going there, so we almost reconciled ourselves to several more years of mutual disagreement and distrust. Then his hockey team went to Harbin, an industrial rust-belt city some 500 miles north of Beijing, to play the Chinese national junior team. 'We were beaten thirteen-nil!' he wailed on his return. 'It could have been worse,' I replied. 'It was,' he said, 'that was just the girls' team. The boys took one look at our performance and decided we were so bad that they didn't think it was worth challenging us.'

Six weeks later Christian and I were on the overnight sleeper to Harbin. He spent the next three months living in an eight-man dormitory with iron bunk beds and straw mattresses, following an ice time schedule that might start as early as 5.45 a.m and finish at midnight. On his arrival he was given two enamel bowls that fitted inside one another, which he would take to the canteen to be filled with food then wash out with cold water in a stone sink. The food was good and plentiful, even if it had to be eaten off formica-topped tables which were usually covered with the remnants of a previous diner's meal.

Christian learnt a lot of Chinese swear words in Harbin, some time-management skills and the importance of wearing long-johns. He told me that in the time he spent in the boarding school he never saw a student take a day sick; a stark comparison to his western friends who, despite, or perhaps because of, their centrally-heated classrooms and school buses, seemed to drop like flies in the winter months. Despite some tough moments, like getting locked outside at night in freezing temperatures for six hours, Christian says that the time he spent in Harbin was the happiest in his life.

Yet the western media gives us a very different picture of where we are likely to find happiness, one that leaves young people in particular with unrealistic expectations. A new car, a new outfit, a holiday in the sun or a box of chocolates are marketed as panaceas. While 'super models' give the subliminal message that super-thin is super-happy, diet plans promise access to super model super happiness.

With so much perfection promised, we become indignant when things don't go our way. When we are ill, for example, we expect the pharmacy or the hospital to deliver a cure rather than reviewing our diet and lifestyle and wondering where we might have gone wrong. Inability to accept one's natural body shape is a major problem in the West, exacerbated, of course, by a badly-balanced diet that does not help the body feel well and quick-fix diet products that do not deliver. My journey in the Taoist way of thinking has led me to believe that every overweight person has a slim body on the inside, and vice versa, which does much to explain the eating disorders and obsessive diet regimes that abound in the West. If your fat person is a threat to you, acknowledge it, relax about your shape and don't be afraid to eat, rather than pushing your whole body with a punishing regime of starvation. If your slim person is the hidden one, let it emerge naturally by nourishing it with foods that will restore the balance in your body.

The wilful deprivation of bodily nourishment that occurs in anorexia is not, psychologists tell us, simply about food. In a period of rapid change, when young people may be buffeted by pressure from peers and parents or under stress academically, they often find themselves unable to strike a balance in their lives, so they try to exert strong control over one particular area. They become unable, or unwilling, to accept that they are getting bigger, so they try to block it out, sometimes causing the mind to lose track of reality. Deprived of nourishment, as the result of an increasingly limited range of foods, they become less and less able to restore the balance they have lost. Thus their *Qi* supply gradually weakens, and the situation, if not checked, can become life-threatening.

Chinese people are able to be more relaxed about the changes that take place in the body over time, because they understand the concept of transformation through the

Five Elements cycle. And they are helped by a diet that satis-
fies their Five Organs and nourishes their *Qi*.

It is ironic that in pursuit of an illusory happiness, often
associated with the perfect image, most people in the West
put themselves under tremendous stress. Stress or worry is the
emotion linked to the spleen and stomach. I have already
explained the damage that we do to these organs by our by
eating habits. Further damage to these organs will lead to more
digestive upsets and increased risk of weight gain – which of
course then causes more stress.

The fifteenth secret of the Chinese food culture is to accept
that life has its ups and downs. There is no absolute good or
absolute bad according to Taoist thought, and this has shaped
the Chinese attitude to life. Thus there is no preference for
success or failure or for the weak or the strong. In fact, in
China, the weak (*yin*) is often respected, as it is the side of
non-violence and peace, as opposed to the strong (*yang*), which
tends to violence and is only in the position of honour during
times of war. Not convinced? A well-known folk story explains
the Chinese mindset much better than I ever could. Sai Weng,
a farmer, had a treasured horse. One day it went missing and
the neighbours offered sympathy. But Sai Weng asked them,
'What makes you think that this is misfortune?' The horse
then returned, bringing several wild companions with it. But
the man refused his neighbours' congratulations, saying, 'What
makes you think that this is good luck?' As the family now
had so many horses, the son took up riding but fell off and
broke his leg. Again, the man refused to see the incident as
misfortune. The following year war broke out and the boy,
because he was lame, was saved from having to go to war.
The Chinese acceptance of the fact that not everybody has a
great time all the time is in stark contrast to the western

approach, where the pursuit of happiness, either by the individual or by society, has propelled philosophical argument. Everything will come full circle in the end, so go with the flow and let your stresses slip away. Your mind, and your body, will be healthier.

When I look back at my diet and my relationship with food before I had the privilege of experiencing Chinese food culture first hand, I could be distressed by the opportunities for enjoying delicious food and nourishing my body that I missed in my youth. But, had I not witnessed the vibrant markets, industrious kitchens and abundant tables as an uninitiated 'foreigner' in *Zhong guo*, the Chinese 'Middle Kingdom', I would not have experienced the joy of discovery or have been able to tell my tale from a perspective that you can share with me.

There are three photos on my kitchen wall, taken in 1995. In the first an old man sits on a cart surrounded by bunches of spring onions too big to lift; on a nearby mat there are heaps of chilies in vibrant reds and greens, and piles of sweet potato, *kudzu* and red radish. On his right is a jam-jar half full of tea, on his left a thick blue overcoat that he would have worn as he pedalled into town with his wares in the chill of the early morning. He wears a hat and thick, red, woolly socks but his top half sports only a thin jacket with a single button, which reveals the dark skin of his toned and muscled stomach. As he smiles for the camera he puts a few wrinkles into his otherwise unblemished skin. It is picture of a happy man.

In the second an old women buys aubergines from a similar trolley, which is parked in a row in a tree-lined street. She has selected three and is perusing the purple heap for a fourth. The young vendor waits patiently as she makes her selection. Business is good as usual. The same people pass through every night to buy fresh vegetables for the evening meal. There is a feeling of activity against a background of tranquillity.

The third photo is of a very young Chinese man. He is riding the bike that pulls his vegetable cart. It is fully loaded with perhaps four times his own weight in fresh produce. He is entering on to a main street where a row of bright yellow taxi cabs line the kerb, ready to move off at any time. He is looking at the camera as if to say, 'What have you noticed? What is it about my vegetables that you find so interesting?' Had I stopped him to try to explain he would not have understood.

I had to go half across the world to find out how what it really means to 'eat one's greens', to learn what comprises a truly balanced way of eating and to appreciate why modern diet and exercise regimes will not help resolve our current dietary crisis. In China, healthy eating and moderate regular exercise are not options, they are a way of life – a balanced life that has helped man live in harmony with nature for thousands of years.

An old Chinese proverb says '*Chi yi qian – zhang yi jian*' ('If we fall into a pit, we will gain in wit'). Perhaps it is time to reassess our approach to health and diet, to look back as well as forward and try once more to live in harmony with the natural world.

In our modern society we have the tools to manage the abundant supply of foods that nature has provided and to eat a wholesome, nutritious and varied diet. If we can direct our energies into achieving this aim, rather than burning calories in the gym or using our free time to attend slimming classes, we would be better for it. Food, good food, eaten in the right way, in the right environment, makes you fit, not fat. If we can understand this and put it into practice I believe that there is hope for us yet and a great deal of enjoyment and many a delicious meal along the way.

Notes

1   Denise Davidson, Azure Dee Welborn Thill and Denise Lash, 'Male and Female Body Shape Preference of Young Children in United States, Mainland China and Turkey', *Child Study Journal*, vol. 32 (2002).

2   Chart extract from T. C. Campbell and T. M. Campbell, *The China Study* (Dallas, TX: Benbella Books, 2005), p. 100.

3   D. Williamson, 'New study shows second generation immigrant children gaining weight', UNC-CH News Services, available online at http://www.unc.edu/news/archives/may98/popkin2.html

4   Author unknown, 'China's appeal for cabbage is withering', *China Daily*, 11 May 2003, available online at http://www.chinadaily.com.cn/en/doc/2003-11/05/content_278697.htm

5   H. Boriss and M. Kreith, 'Commodity Profile: Cabbage' (Agricultural Marketing Resource Center, University of California, 2006.)

6   E. N. Anderson, *The Food of China* (New Haven and London: Yale University Press, 1998), *notes* table 1.

7   P. Clayton, *Health Defence*, 2nd edn (Aylesbury: Accelerated Learning Systems, 2004), p. 217.

8   Five-spice is actually a generic term used to cover a mixture that can vary in content (and number of spices) but which usually includes star anise, Sichuan peppercorns, cassia (Chinese cinnamon), cloves and fennel.

9   'What every consumer should know about Trans Fatty Acids' (9 July 2003), U.S Food and Drug Administration Fact Sheet.

10   R. Fletcher and K. Fairfield, 'Vitamins for Chronic Disease Prevention in Adults', *JAMA*, vol. 287, no. 23 (June 2002).

11   Campbell and Campbell, op.cit., p. 74.

12   Clayton, *Health Defence*, op.cit., p. 95.

13   Ibid., p. 251.

14   Henry C. Lu's *Chinese System of Food Cures* is extremely informative on the *yin* and *yang* values of foods and their suitability for different body types (see Further Reading).

15   A Chinese philosopher of the third century BC and interpreter of Confucius. He believed in the innate goodness of human nature.

16   D. Yi, P. Yong, L. Wenkui, *Chinese Functional Food* (Beijing: New World Press, 1999), p. 99.

17   Herbert A Giles, trans., *Chuang Tzu XV*, p. 192.

18   A. Parker and N. Dagnall, *Effects of Bilateral Eye Movements on Gist False Recognition in the DRM Paradigm, Brain and Cognition*, vol. 63, no. 3 (April 2007) available online at http://www.science direct.com.

19   P. H. Lahmann, C. Friedenreich *et al.*, 'Physical Activity and Breast Cancer Risk: The European Prospective Investigation into Cancer and Nutrition' in *Cancer Epidemiology Biomarkers & Prevention* 16 (January 2007) available online at http://www.cebp.aacrjournals.org: 36–42.

Further reading

Anderson, E. N, *The Food of China* (New Haven and London: Yale University Press, 1998).

Bredon, J. and I. Mitrophanow, *The Moon Year* (Shanghai: Kelly and Walsh, 1927).

Campbell, T. C. and T. M. Campbell, *The China Study* (Dallas, TX: Benbella Book, 2005).

Clayton, P., *Health Defence* (Aylesbury: Accelerated Learning Systems Ltd., 2004).

Cooper, J. C., *Taoism: The Way of the Mystic* (London: Mandala, 1991).

Chang, K.C., *Food in Chinese Culture: Anthropological and Historical Perspectives* (Taipei: SMC Publishing, 1997).

Dunlop, F., *Sichuan Food* (London: Michael Joseph, 2001).

Fullerton-Smith, J., *The Truth about Food* (London: Bloomsbury Publishing, 2007).

Jingfeng, B., *Episodes in Traditional Chinese Medicine*, trans. Z. Tingquan (Beijing: Panda Books, Chinese Literature Press, 1998).

Jingfeng, C., *Eating Your Way to Health: Dietotherapy in Traditional Chinese Medicine* (Beijing: Foreign Languages Press, 1988).

Larkcom, J., *Oriental Vegetables: The Complete Guide for the Gardening Cook* (London: John Murray, 1998).

Lau, D. C., trans., *Confucius: The Analects (Lun Yu)* (Hong Kong: The Chinese University Press, 1992).

Lu, H. C., *Chinese System of Food Cures* (New York: Sterling Publishing Co., 1986).

———, *Chinese Herbs with Common Foods* (Tokyo: Kondansha International, 1997).

Maoshing, N. I., trans., *The Yellow Emperor's Classic of Medicine (Neijing Suwen)* (Boston and London: Shambhala, 1995).

Mitscher, L. A and V. Dolby, *The Green Tea Book: China's Fountain of Youth* (New York: Avery Publishing, 1998).

Ody, P., *Practical Chinese Medicine* (New Delhi: New Age Books, 2003).

Porter Smith. F and Stuart. G.A., trans. *Chinese Medicinal Herbs (Li Shih-Chen).* Mineola, New York: Dover Publications, 2003)

Reichstein, G., *Wood Becomes Water: Chinese Medicine in Everyday Life* (New York, Tokyo and London: Kondansha International, 1998).

Shurtleff, W. and A. Aoyagi, *The Book of Tofu* (Berkeley, CA: Ten Speed Press, 2001).

Shou-zhong. Y., trans. *The Divine Farmer's Materia Medica* (Boulder, Co: Blue Poppy Press, 1998).

So, Y.-K., *Classic Food of China* (London: Macmillan, 1994).

Spencer, C., *British Food: An Extraordinary Thousand Years of History* (London: Grub Street, 2004).

Stitt. P. A. *Fighting the Food Giants.* (Manitowoc: Natural Press, 1981).

Tsuei, W., *Roots of Chinese Culture and Medicine* (Malaysia: Pelanduk Publications, 1992).

Williams, T., *Chinese Medicine* (London: Vega, 2002).

Zhao, Z. and G. Ellis, *The Healing Cuisine of China: 300 recipes for Vibrant Health and Longevity* (Vermont: Healing Arts Press, 1998).

Yi, D., P. Yong and L. Wenkui, *Chinese Functional Food* (Beijing: New World Press, 1999).

Wu, J. C. H., trans., *Tao Te Ching* (Boston and London: Shambala, 2006).